D1564678

WHAT AILS THE WHITE HOUSE

An Introduction to the Medical History of the American Presidency

By

Jay W. Murphy, M.D.

Cover photo: *President Garfield in sickbed in the White House in 1881.* Courtesy of the Library of Congress Prints & Photographs.

ISBN: 978-1-58597-398-9

Library of Congress Control Number: 2006928710

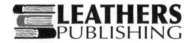

LEATHERS
PUBLISHING

A division of Squire Publishers, Inc.
4500 College Blvd.
Overland Park, KS 66211
1/888/888-7696
www.leatherspublishing.com

*Dedicated to my wife, Robin —
my life's companion, best friend
and greatest blessing.*

RICHARD G. LUGAR
INDIANA

306 HART SENATE OFFICE BUILDING
WASHINGTON, DC 20510
202–224–4814

senator_lugar@lugar.senate.gov

COMMITTEES:
FOREIGN RELATIONS, CHAIRMAN
AGRICULTURE, NUTRITION, AND FORESTRY

United States Senate

WASHINGTON, DC 20510–1401

May 1, 2006

Dear Dr. Murphy:

Thank you for sending me a working copy of *What Ails the White House*. I appreciate the opportunity to provide the following written endorsement of your excellent book:

In *What Ails the White House: A Primer on the Medical History of the American Presidency*, Dr. Jay Murphy provides the reader with a compelling account of the physical health of the 43 U.S. presidents. Drawing upon his decades of experience in cardiology and an impressive knowledge of American history, Dr. Murphy examines the ailments that have befallen American presidents, the treatment they have received, and the ensuing consequences for the White House and American politics.

Dr. Murphy's research includes fascinating accounts of White House medical events that are not well-known -- covered-up heart attacks, a secret surgery on a private yacht, and even self-bleedings. By focusing on some of the most worrisome moments of American presidencies, Dr. Murphy's scholarship offers a unique testament to the durability of American democracy: even during times of dire medical emergency in the White House, the presidency and our nation have continued to function with extraordinary stability.

Beyond its valuable contributions to presidential history, this work highlights the incredible progress that has been made in science and medicine since George Washington's time, when, as Dr. Murphy notes, it was no small feat to simply reach the age of thirty five -- the minimum age of eligibility for the presidency.

I wish you the best of luck with publication and thank you, again, for contacting me.

Sincerely,

Richard G. Lugar
United States Senator

RGL/msd

ABOUT THE BOOK

AMERICANS HAVE ALWAYS been keenly interested in the medical problems of the rich and famous. This is no less the case with the medical illnesses of our presidents. Dr. Jay Murphy has now provided us with a well-documented, authoritative and appropriately detailed, yet concise treatise on the medical problems of our presidents.

There are several examples of serious illness being withheld from the press and in many instances willful obfuscation of the facts.

- Grover Cleveland's oral cancer surgery while on a yacht, with the press informed that he had a tooth extraction.

- Woodrow Wilson's incapacitating stroke that resulted in his wife carrying out the duties of president.

- Franklin Delano Roosevelt re-elected in 1940 with severe hypertension and congestive heart failure, diagnoses his cardiologist was not permitted to discuss.

- John F. Kennedy's Addison's disease (adrenal insufficiency) was evident from a careful reading of the *American Medical Association Archives of Surgery* in 1955, well before his presidential campaign of 1960.

Current candidates for major elected office are usually asked to disclose their medical histories. Major newspapers analyze and detail in lay terms any medical problems so identified.

Consider the press coverage of Ronald Reagan after he was shot in 1981. Every key event from the emergency room, to surgery, to recovery and discharge was well detailed and is captured in Dr. Murphy's account of these events.

Dr. Murphy's book is skillfully done, and it is one of those books where if one starts reading it, one cannot put it down. It is a fascinating account of White House events and underscores the tremendous progress in health care in the last century. It is a very good read and can be enjoyed by non-physicians as well as physicians.

— Norton J. Greenberger, M.D.
Clinical Professor of Medicine
Harvard Medical School

ACKNOWLEDGMENTS

LIVING WITH ME is no bargain and becomes less so when I am engrossed in a creative project. So first and foremost, my love, thanks, appreciation and admiration go to Robin, my wife, who had to endure a litany of ideas, moods and midnight inspirations during the writing of this book. Without her steadfast, unconditional love, support and clear counsel, this book would never have been written. She is truly one of God's angels.

Thanks to my children, Matthew and Megan, for their love, support and review of this book. I love you both and am proud and blessed beyond words to be your father.

I would like to thank Jack E. Wingate, James A. Byrnes, William B. Toalson, M.D., Jay R. Richardson, M.D., and Brian M. Friedman, M.D., for review of early iterations of this text and for their suggestions and encouragement.

Special appreciation to my partners at Cardiology Services, Drs. Thomas Baldwin, Steven Whitfield, Brian Friedman, Richard Brown, David Rios, Rangarao Tummala, William Emmot, Kit Powers, Steven Obermueller, Patrick Santiago, Murali Muppala, Timothy Beaver and James Marcum, and also the administration of Olathe Health Systems Inc. who allow me the time to pursue other interests, secure in the knowledge that my patients will always receive the best care.

I greatly appreciate the research assistance of the library staffs of both Olathe Medical Center and Shawnee Mission Medical Center and the superb editing of Maria Goodier.

I do not consider myself an author, rather an individual with a vocational interest in medicine and recreational interest in presidential history. This dissertation originates from an oral presentation initially prepared for fellow physicians and health care workers at "Heartbeat 2004" conference in Olathe, Kansas, with subsequent lectures in the Kansas City area. If not for the multiple individuals with the post-presentation suggestion of "You should write I book," I would never have conquered my personal insecurities or inertia to write this text. Thank you for your kindness and encouragement. I hope this manuscript meets or exceeds your expectations.

TABLE OF CONTENTS

PROLOGUE

SINCE ITS INCEPTION of the presidency in 1789, America has had 43 presidents, 42 different men, men different in many ways — politics, political parties, personalities, leadership styles, education, wealth, social status and geographic origins. Volumes explore these distinct and individual characteristics in minute detail and theorize regarding the historical implications of these presidential dissimilarities. But an undeniably shared trait has received less scrutiny. All presidents have been human, mortal and, therefore, susceptible to the same illnesses, maladies and injuries as the rest of mankind. Though the presidents often seem, in the public conscience, larger than life and immune to the woes of ordinary human beings, in fact, the presidency renders American presidents more susceptible to bodily injury during White House years than at any other time of their lives. This is largely due to the occupational hazard of assassination. Another dichotomy exists. Although elected presidents to the present time have been exclusively men and mostly over 50 years of age, a category of the population in which disability is common, no elected president has ever relinquished the office for longer than a few hours for health reasons.

For me, as a physician, the study of the illnesses of the American presidents holds a fascination because it intermingles the evolution of several separate histories. It starts, of course, with the history of the illnesses or injuries that presidents have endured, especially while in office. What were they? What was the causation and what diagnostic and treatment options were available to the presidents and medical practitioners of the time? We would presume and hope that American presidents, the leader of our country and today the leader of the free world, through all eras would have received the best medical care available. But is this verified by history?

As opposed to illness in the general population, presidential ailments have political consequences. Presidential incapability or disability, which has been present but not acknowledged at several times in history, or death caused by illness and injury affects the dominant branch of the federal government of the United States, the executive branch. This, in turn, may impact or influence United States history as well as world history. After all, the American president is referred to as the "most powerful man on the face of the earth." What have been the political consequences of presidential illness/injury and how may American or world history have varied if the illnesses had been prevented or differently treated?

Surgical and medical capabilities change vastly by the decade. Medicine today is unrecognizable compared to the limited and often harmful remedies employed by physicians at the dawn of the American presidency. George Washington pleaded with his doctors to allow him to die with dignity after the torture of his physicians' treatments which would be considered barbaric today. Previously fatal illnesses are now routinely cured, if not prevented altogether. Could 21st century medicine, if somehow miraculously available to earlier presidents, have prevented presidential illnesses and ultimately impacted or altered history? We would hope that history may have been influenced constructively. But what assumptions can be made from the medical and historical facts available?

As the "most powerful man on the face of the earth," the president has the very best of American medicine available to him. The choice of the president's personal physician rests with the president. Have presidents chosen their physician wisely and have those physicians served their patrons skillfully?

Also, we would hope that the officials of the administrations of stricken presidents would discharge duty with the best interest of the country at heart. But administrative officials owe allegiance to the president, who appointed them. The power and prestige of their positions is derived only from their service to a president. If the president is no longer in office, whether by illness, death or other vagaries, their influence evaporates. Human nature being what it is, one might expect disinclination under these circumstances to altruistically place the nation's interest before self-interest. Indeed, this appears verified by history. Presidential illness reveals a pattern of misrepresentation or concealment of presidential medical information from the public. Ill presidents have been surrounded by willing minions, even surrogates, who have conspired to protect power before principles. Much of the hidden illness in the White House occurred in the 19th century or first half of the 20th century, before the emergence of the American media as we know it today. One could persuasively argue that the media's growth and maturation as the watchdog of the president and entire political process exceeds even the changes in American medicine. Could illness be effectively hidden today? What have been the overall effects of the American media on the American presidency and the political process? The effects on the disclosure of presidential illness and image of presidential health are remarkable and intriguing. We would hope that open access to and greater accountability of presidential administrations may have improved government. Surprisingly, viewed through the microscope of history, this expectation indeed may be verified.

Please enjoy *What Ails the White House: An Introduction to the Health of the American Presidency.*

CHAPTER 1

The Early Presidents

Early Health Hazards

The Constitution stipulates a person must be 35 years of age or older to become president of the United States. Attaining this age was no meager accomplishment in the 18th and 19th centuries. In fact, the mean survival age at the time of George Washington's birth in the 1730s was approximately 35 years. Infant mortality, death in the first year of life, alone approached 50 percent and contributed significantly to this low

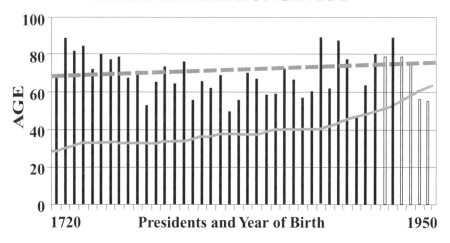

PRESIDENTIAL LONGEVITY

The estimated year of birth of the presidents is displayed along the horizontal axis. Vertical bars indicate the age at death of the individual presidents. Living presidents are represented by light bars and deceased presidents by dark bars. The grey line represents the mean age of survival which has risen dramatically over the 200 years of the American presidency. The dotted line approximates the estimated survival (assuming good health) at the time of presidential inauguration.

survival age. Survival to young adulthood portended a better lifespan than suggested by mean survival alone.

Compared to the 21st century, the populace in the 18th century confronted enormous health obstacles. Sanitation systems were primitive, water purification unknown. A drink of water could germinate a life-threatening or fatal disease. Open hearths furnished heat, but also polluted the air and promoted respiratory illnesses. Contaminated or spoiled foods were a constant threat. Every bite of food potentially threatened one's life. If one became ill, most medical treatments, by our current knowledge, worsened the illness.

No antibiotics existed. Complications of simple infections such as a cut or blister could result in death. Currently curable afflictions such as pneumonia were usually fatal illnesses. Immunizations were primitive or did not exist, and epidemics of smallpox and cholera could devastate and kill 25 to 60 percent of a population. Surgical and obstetrical practices were very limited. Pregnancy, with its high infant and maternal mortality, was best considered a disease rather than a blessed event.

With all these environmental and medical impediments, the first seven presidents remarkably lived to an average age of nearly 80 years old. The nascent republic of the United States of America did not experience disabling or fatal diseases to presidents in the White House for the first 60 years of its existence. Eight presidents have died in the White House in the subsequent 160 years, an average of one death each 20 years, and several other presidents have been disabled for varying lengths of time. Whether the struggling nation, torn by the issues of slavery, sovereignty of states rights vs. federal jurisdiction and general mistrust of centralized and remote government, could have survived instability in the executive branch due to illness or disability is problematic.

Overall, the American presidents have been a group of survivors compared to their peers (light line, Table 1). Even as mean survival rate has risen, average presidential survival exceeds the mean. Occasional exceptions are seen, often due to the occupational hazard of assassination. With four living former presidents, three exceeding 80 years of age, the survival advantage for presidents seems unlikely to change soon.

Still, some authors suggest that the presidency is a life-shortening experience. This theory is based on actuarial tables for life expectancy

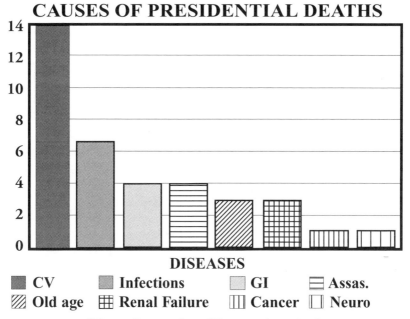

CAUSES OF PRESIDENTIAL DEATHS

DISEASES

■ CV ■ Infections ☐ GI ≡ Assas.
▨ Old age ⊞ Renal Failure ⦀ Cancer ⊡ Neuro

CV=cardiovascular; GI=gastrointestinal.

at the age the presidents entered office (dotted line, Table 1). Comparative survival by this analysis, not including living or assassinated presidents, is more near the average of the general population.

To suggest a survival disadvantage by this analysis ignores the fact that actuarial estimation of life expectancy assumes good health at the time of the estimate. As outlined in this text, several presidents were unhealthy, if not fatally ill, when elected and would not qualify, if submitted to the intense scrutiny of an insurance underwriter, as healthy subjects when entering office.

The causes of death of the American presidents are similar to the general population. Cardiovascular diseases[1] account for nearly 50 per-

---

[1] Cardiovascular diseases are caused by atherosclerosis, which may involve the arteries to the heart, brain or legs most commonly, but potentially the arteries to any organ of the body. Atherosclerosis begins with the deposition of lipoproteins, a combination of fats and proteins that normally circulate in the blood, into the wall of the artery. The lipoprotein rich in cholesterol, low density lipoprotein (LDL), is the main culprit. Over a period of years deposition leads to obstruction of the arteries, which can result in heart attacks, strokes or shortage of blood supply to the legs. Recent evidence indicates that thrombosis, the formation of a *(cont. next page)*

cent of deaths in America in the 21st century. Cardiovascular disease is also the leading cause of death in the American presidents, claiming the lives of 14 of the 37 deceased presidents. The percentage of deaths due to cardiovascular disease lags that of the general population probably because many presidents succumbed to infections in an era before antibiotics and four presidents (11 percent) have suffered a violent death due to assassination. This is a percentage that far exceeds the public risk of traumatic death. These statistics emphasize that assassination is, indeed, an occupational hazard of the American presidency.

Those that postulate the stress of the American presidency contributes to a shortened life span point out that presidential survival lags survival of male members of Congress and the Supreme Court, groups with similar educational and socio-economic backgrounds. Whereas others render collective decisions, the presidency demands singular judgments, and this unique position of power also targets the office as the focal point of national controversies.

Scientific studies suggest that personality type, if not stress, is associated with an increased risk of cardiovascular diseases. The so-called Type A personality individual, who is driven, goal-oriented and hyperreactive to stress, anxiety, anger and fear, is most at risk. This is the likely personality type of individuals able to successfully scale the political mountain to the presidential summit. Less clearly and more controversially, stress also may impact the immune system, rendering stressed individuals more susceptible to infections and malignancies.

---

blood clot at the site of bodily injury, contributes to atherosclerosis and clinical events as well. Sites of atherosclerosis, even if not severe enough to occlude blood supply, can activate the clotting system of the circulating blood, causing occlusion of vessels by clot within the vessel.

Atherosclerosis of the abdominal aorta can lead to expansion of the aortic wall, aneurysm formation, and eventually, much like an overinflated balloon, rupture with life-threatening internal bleeding.

Health features related to the development of atherosclerosis (risk factors) have been identified and include high cholesterol levels, high blood pressure, diabetes, smoking, sedentary life style and a family history of vascular disease. Control of risk factors, either by diet, lifestyle change or medications can greatly reduce the probability of vascular disease or, in those with established atherosclerosis, reduce the likelihood of suffering a clinical event such as heart attack or stroke.

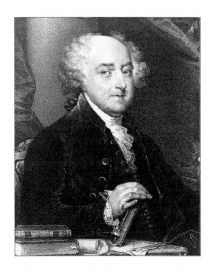 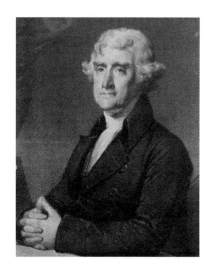

John Adams (left), the second president of the United States, and Thomas Jefferson (right), the third president of the United States. Courtesy of the Library of Congress Prints and Photographs.

To me, the intrigue and interest of illness and the American presidency is not whether the presidency has induced illness, but rather how illness, when it has occurred, has affected the function and effectiveness of the presidents and the executive branch of government. Ill presidents have generally been ineffective presidents, and deceased presidents are replaced by vice presidents often with markedly different agendas and politics. So ultimately, disease has affected American and world history.

One quirk of fate regarding the early presidents is worthy of note. John Adams, the second president of the United States and a member of the Federalist Party, and Thomas Jefferson, the third president of the United States and a member of the Democratic-Republican Party, were political rivals and philosophical opposites throughout their careers.[2]

In their long retirements, they were cordial correspondents via letter, but still polar opposites in political views. Adams, at age 91, and Jefferson, at age 83, both died on the same day in 1826. Adams, who was the

---

[2] The Constitution did not anticipate political parties. Indeed, they were considered an anathema in colonial times. But inevitably differences in interpretation of the Constitution and implementation of governmental policies led to political factions and eventually to the two-party system. These differences began *(cont. next page)*

president with the longest life span until recently eclipsed by Ronald Reagan, died in Massachusetts. Reportedly, his final words were, "Jefferson still survives." He did not know that Jefferson had expired several hours earlier in Virginia. The day was July 4, 1826, the 50th anniversary of the signing of the Declaration of Independence and the birth of the United States. Fate allowed both men to honor the birth of the nation to which they dedicated their lives with the timing of their deaths.

Andrew Jackson

A great example of the health obstacles and hardships facing the early presidents is the medical history of Andrew Jackson. His physical status throughout his life belied his mental strength and personal courage. He was thin of stature, almost cadaverous in appearance. Although six feet in height, his adult weight never exceeded 145 pounds. He was cocky, temperamental, argumentative, opinionated and competitive. These personality traits contributed to his medical conditions. In an era

during Washington's tenure as president. Adams, the first vice president, favored an aristocratic form of government administered by men of property. He supported federal sovereignty over states' rights, and the establishment of a National Bank. He also favored cooperation and alliance with the British rather than the French. Jefferson, the first secretary of state, best summarized his politics in the Declaration of Independence, which he authored: "We hold these truths to be self-evident, that all men are created equal, that they are endowed by their Creator with certain unalienable Rights, that among these are Life, Liberty and the pursuit of Happiness." He favored a more inclusive participation in the political process, and championed the participation of all men, whether property owners or not, in the political process. He favored local government and states' rights over an omnipotent federal government and favored treaties with the French rather than the British. These differences caused much discord in Washington's administration and eventually caused Jefferson to resign his post as secretary of state.

Formation of political factions and the lack of anticipation of same by the Constitution made for strange bedfellows in early administrations. The Constitution stipulated that the second-place finisher in electoral votes for the office of president became the vice president. Thus Jefferson, who opposed Adams for the presidency in 1796, became vice president when Adams became president as the Constitution mandated.

Historians argue that the two-party system, by forcing a wide range of political opinions into two coalitions, standardizes a method of dissent, and has thus been a major contributor to the success of our republican form of government.

with no modern medicine or surgery, it is a miracle that the belligerent Jackson survived to become the seventh president of the United States. But his indomitable will allowed him to conquer many obstacles and overcome his own health maladies.

Jackson was born in the Waxhaw settlement in the Carolinas in 1767. When the Revolutionary War commenced, Jackson was 13 years old and still too small to lug a musket. Therefore, he volunteered as messenger for the Continental Army troops. Jackson and his brother were captured by British forces. Shortly after his capture, the young Jackson was ordered by a British officer to clean the soldier's boots. Jackson, not one to be bullied into menial tasks, replied, "I am a prisoner of war and claim to be treated as such." Infuriated, the British officer struck a saber blow at Jackson, inflicting deep gashes on the boy's forehead and left hand, which scarred Jackson for life.

Jackson and his brother were then marched 40 miles (from modern-day North Carolina into South Carolina) and thrown into a prison. They received no bedding, medicine, dressings or medical attention for their wounds. Both Jacksons contracted smallpox while in prison, a disease epidemic during the Revolutionary War.[3]

Fortunately, Jackson's mother arrived just as an exchange of British and American prisoners occurred and persuaded authorities to include her sons in the exchange. Jackson returned the 40 miles home to North Carolina with his mother and brother, barefoot and without a jacket, with festering sword wounds and smallpox. His brother died shortly after arriving home. Andrew survived after days of fever and delirium, and a long convalescence.

Jackson was orphaned at age 15 at the death of his mother, a nurse who died while tending injured soldiers. He migrated with relatives to Tennessee. Historians agree Jackson survived multiple brawls on the

---

[3] Two-thirds of the American casualties of the Revolutionary War were due to illness rather than combat. Smallpox was epidemic among the troops and claimed over 100,000 lives. George Washington was immune because of childhood exposure to the disease. Washington strongly supported inoculation to prevent the disease at a time when the medical community largely opposed it. Some historians claim Washington's implementation of a mandatory inoculation program for the Continental Army was his most important strategic decision during his military career.

Tennessee frontier, but two clearly affected his health.

In 1806 Jackson challenged a Charles Dickinson to a duel when the latter, legend has it, insulted the honor of Jackson's wife, Rachel. Unfortunately for Jackson, Mr. Dickinson was an excellent marksman. Unfortunately for Dickinson, even his marksmanship was no match for the stout constitution of Andrew Jackson.

The duel took place at 10 paces. Apparently the slender Jackson wore a very large coat, making it more difficult for Dickinson to precisely locate Jackson's torso as his target. Dickinson fired first, striking Jackson in the chest. Jackson briefly staggered and grabbed his chest. He was able to recover, then aim and fire his own weapon. He inflicted a painful wound to Dickinson's pelvis which proved fatal by nightfall. Jackson staggered from the dueling field, the victor, but with his own blood filling and overflowing his boots and spilling to the ground. Remembering the duel, Jackson stated, "I should have hit him, if he had shot me through the brain." This testament became part of the lore that forged Jackson's national image.

Now, mind you, from a medical standpoint, we do not have subsequent X-rays, CT scans, intensive care unit records or daily physician notes documenting Jackson's gunshot wound, but Jackson's health was never the same after the duel. Although he survived the initial hemorrhage, he had a lifelong persistent cough, intermittent purulent (infected) sputum production and intermittent, life-threatening pulmonary hemorrhages (bleeding from the lungs). Often chills, fever and profuse sweats would accompany these episodes. Physician biographers suspect that Dickinson's bullet lodged in Jackson's chest and initiated a chronic infection. A lung abscess[4] initiated from dust, clothing or other foreign material entering the chest with the bullet or chronic bronchitis and bronchiestasis[5], due to partial obstruction by the bullet of a major bronchus (airway) with resulting infection and destruction of the bronchi, are both possibilities and may have co-existed. Recurrent pulmonary

---

[4] Lung abscess is a localized cavity of infection within the lung.

[5] Bronchiectasis is irreversible, focal bronchial (airway) dilation due to destruction of the elastic and muscular components of the bronchial wall, usually caused by chronic infection.

hemorrhages left Jackson anemic and near death several times through-out his life.

A second altercation, a street brawl in 1812, involved the Benton brothers, the ancestors of Thomas Hart Benton, a famous Missouri art-ist. In the melee, Jackson was shot, receiving a ball which shattered his left shoulder joint. Attending physicians recommended amputation of his left arm, but Jackson refused. Although the arm was saved, it was of little functional use thereafter and the source of chronic pain and likely osteomyelitis.[6]

Just over a month after the Benton shooting incident, duty called. Jackson, the commander of the Tennessee militia, with a fresh wound and arm in sling, led the troops to border war battles with various Indian tribes of the American frontier and eventually to battles with the British in the War of 1812. These military campaigns took a great physical toll on Jackson. His shoulder wound continued to fester, and small pieces of bone worked their way to the skin surface. Jackson included these bone shards in his letters home to his wife. Jackson developed both dysen-tery[7] and malaria,[8] diseases commonly afflicting the soldiers in mili-tary campaigns of that era.

Wracked with pain, besieged by fevers, seized with bouts of ab-dominal pain and dysentery causing up to 30 stools in a 12-hour period, Jackson endured, allowing no surrender in either himself or his men. At one point Jackson faced a mutiny of his own soldiers and threatened to shoot the first soldier to break ranks. The soldiers all returned to their

---

[6] Osteomyelitis is the inflammation and destruction of bone caused by infection. This can occur at the site of bone penetrated by trauma or frequently in diabetics with extension of skin infections to bone. Treatment requires prolonged intrave-nous antibiotic administration.

[7] Dysentery is an intestinal inflammation characterized by bloody diarrhea and ab-dominal pain. Amebiasis, a parasitic infection of the bowel caused by ingestion of contaminated drinking water, was the most likely cause of Jackson's symptoms. Amoebae are one-celled organisms present in most rivers and streams.

[8] Malaria is a chronic parasitic infection causing periodic paroxysms of chills, fever, sweats and anemia. It is carried by and contracted through bites of the anophelene mosquito.

starving and pestilent positions rather than test Jackson's will. But at other times Jackson was known to give up his horse to a wounded soldier. Jackson was a natural commander and earned the moniker of "Old Hickory" from his men for his strength, courage and leadership.

Jackson gained national recognition with his victory at the Battle of New Orleans in 1815, the last battle of the War of 1812 against the British. It's important to recall national pride had been sorely bruised by the fall and subsequent burning of Washington, D.C. by British troops early in the War of 1812. President Madison had been forced to evacuate from the White House during this phase of the war.

Actually, the Treaty of Ghent ending the War of 1812 was signed by negotiating diplomats in Europe two weeks before the Battle of New Orleans occurred. But in an era with no telephones, telegraphs, let alone e-mail, faxes and satellite communications, word of the treaty had not reached the battle lines. The victory at the Battle of New Orleans was aided by the death of the commanding British general early in the battle. The American flag flew over the battlefield at the end of the day. Jackson's military victory against the British electrified the nation and restored Union pride. Jackson became a national hero.

After additional campaigns in Florida against the Seminole Indians, campaigns accompanied by recurrence of fevers and dysentery, and a brief stint as the appointed governor of the Florida Territory, Jackson finally returned home to Tennessee. He was physically exhausted, in poor health and in need of a well-deserved rest. But already political forces were urging Jackson's participation in national politics. Rachel, Jackson's wife, was opposed to any political career for Jackson, stating to a niece, "He is not a well man and never will be unless they allow him to rest." Even Jackson demurred initially, stating, "Do they think that I am such a damned fool as to think myself fit for president of the United States? No, sir; I know what I am fit for. I can command a body of men in a rough way, but I am not fit to be president."

Jackson benefited from a changing American electorate. Up to that time only men owning property had been allowed to vote, and thus elected representatives tended to be from the American aristocracy. But in 1824 when Jackson first ran for president, state election laws were morphing and allowing the laboring masses to vote. Elections were rau-

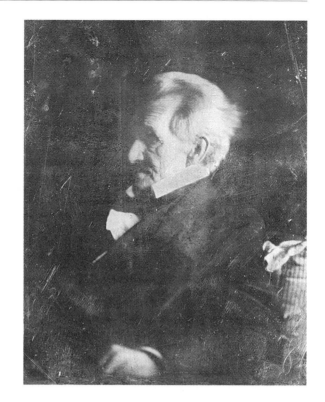

Andrew Jackson, the seventh president of the United States late in life (circa 1845). Courtesy of Library of Congress Prints and Photographs.

cous affairs with no shortage of hard cider. Compared to other candidates, Jackson was a man of the common people with his frontier heritage and military leadership. Jackson also may have benefited from the campaigning mores of the time. Candidates would graciously agree to allow their names to be placed before the electorate but it was undignified for a man to appear to be seeking the office of president of the United States. Candidates did not attend the nominating convention or stump for votes on the campaign trail. Campaigning was a job for the candidate's supporters and minions, not for the candidate himself. When elected, a "humble" candidate would accept his nation's "call to duty." Jackson's health would not have allowed him to travel for prolonged periods. Campaigning would have been out of the question. If he lived in a different era, I wonder what an odiferous impression Jackson may have made on the electorate with his combination of purulent sputum, pulmonary hemorrhages, osteomyelitis and chronic dysentery.

In the 1824 presidential election, Jackson received a plurality but not a majority of the electoral votes. He lost the presidency by a vote in the House of Representatives to John Quincy Adams. Adams, who finished second in the general election, struck the so-called "corrupt bargain" with Henry Clay, who ran third in the popular vote. Clay threw his support to Adams, and subsequently Clay was appointed secretary of state by President Adams. Both Adams and Clay considered the wilderness-schooled Jackson essentially illiterate, almost barbaric and certainly not fit for the office of president.

Jackson was incensed by the backroom politics and may have launched a successful campaign in the House of Representatives if not felled by a severe pulmonary hemorrhage which left him anemic, bedridden and near death. He could not journey to Washington, D.C. to construct his case. It did not help that his attending physicians treated his pulmonary hemorrhages with blood-letting, which further exacerbated Jackson's anemia.

In 1828, the public, remembering the "corrupt bargain," elected Andrew Jackson as the seventh president of the United States. In a quirk of fate, his beloved Rachel, the devoted wife who discouraged a political career for Jackson in order to protect his health, died from what medical historians believe was a heart attack shortly before the couple was scheduled to depart Tennessee for Washington, D.C. Rachel was buried on Christmas Eve 1828, attired in the gown she had purchased to wear for the inauguration. "My heart is nearly broken," mourned Jackson. Indeed, he grieved Rachel's death throughout his life and remained a widower. Overcoming emotional as well as chronic physical frailties, Jackson traveled to Washington, D.C. and assumed office in 1829. He was re-elected in 1832.

The presidency also was not conducive to Jackson's health. He continued to have recurrent pulmonary hemorrhages. Jackson learned to anticipate an attack of pulmonary hemorrhage and established his own home remedy. He would bare his arm, take his pocket knife, lance his antecubital vein (vein in the bend of the elbow) and bleed himself. He often self-administered this procedure at night in the White House. Shortly after becoming president, he began developing edema (swelling or fluid retention), probably due to congestive heart failure and/or kidney failure, a process which continued and worsened throughout his life.

Jackson was also the first American president attacked with the intent to kill. During his second term a young man fired from point-blank range at President Jackson with two different handguns. In both instances the pistol caps exploded but failed to ignite the powder in the gun barrel and thus failed to discharge the ball. Firearm experts have estimated the chances of a dual misfire of the type of firearms used to be in the range of one in 10,000. Once again the Jackson will or luck prevailed and he was uninjured.

Twenty years after his shoulder wound, when Jackson was the president, pain from this injury became excruciating. Surgery to remove the bullet was performed in the White House. Using the anesthesia of the day, a couple of shots of brandy, an incision was made as Jackson gripped his walking stick. Apparently, the bullet had worked its way from the shoulder joint to a subcutaneous location as the bullet popped out with a relatively superficial skin incision. Extraction of the bullet relieved Jackson's pain from this wound.

Still, Jackson was in constant pain, severely debilitated and certainly incapacitated several times during his eight years as president. During the last three months of his term, he rarely could rise from bed and remained primarily secluded on the second floor of the White House.

But Jackson with all his medical maladies not only survived his presidency, he transformed the presidency. Up until that time, the president had been more of a figurehead position, somewhat like the British monarchy of our time. It was considered the role of Congress to govern and legislate, and the president did not play a large role in policy formation. In the nearly 40 years of the presidency prior to Jackson, the presidential veto had only been used a handful of times and then only if a bill was considered unconstitutional by the vetoing president. Jackson, as stated by the constitution, considered the president the "direct representative of the American people." After all, the president is the office elected by the vote of all the people. He considered it his duty as president to carry out the public will. He believed a president could veto a bill for any reason, constitutional, political, social or economic, and his generous use of the presidential veto greatly expanded the role of the presidency in shaping policy. Thus began a shift of power in the federal government. The president and executive branch of American government became dominant rather than Congress and the legislative branch of government. In the age of video media, one could argue that a transition of power toward the presidency and the executive branch of the federal government continues through our time.

Surprisingly, Jackson survived his presidency and an additional seven years. He died at the age of 77 at his home, The Hermitage, in Tennessee. His last years were grisly, as he developed progressive edema and anasarca (total body swelling due to fluid accumulation). Jackson's self-description was, "I am blubber of water." Certainly, his terminal symptoms were consistent with congestive heart failure, if not kidney failure and liver failure.

An interesting and plausible theory advanced by Dr. Francis Gardner, a physician biographer of Jackson, suggests Jackson's terminal kidney, liver and heart failure may have been caused by secondary amyloidosis. Amyloidosis is a disease marked by an accumulation of insoluble proteins in various internal organs such as the heart, liver and kidneys in amounts sufficient to impair the normal function of those organs. Secondary amyloidosis usually occurs in response to chronic infection. Certainly with two chronic suppurating infections, i.e. bronchiectasis and osteomyelitis, both initiated by bullet wounds, Andrew Jackson's life history suggests he was ripe, so to speak, for this disease.

Finally, some medical experts have suggested that Andrew Jackson may have suffered from heavy metal poisoning because he ingested calomel (mercurous chloride) and sugar of lead (lead acetate) solutions (see footnote 11, page 21) liberally throughout his life. These agents were the anti-inflammatory drugs of Jackson's day. To test this hypothesis, samples of Jackson's hair still extant were analyzed for heavy metal content. The results were published in the *Journal of the American Medical Association* on August 11, 1999. Both mercury and lead levels were elevated in the Jackson hair samples, indicating exposure, possibly even low level lead toxicity. However, levels did not approach the lethal range to suggest death due to heavy metal poisoning.

Jackson's medical history is an example of the hardiness, stoicism and stamina characteristic of many presidents. Those who became ill, necessarily highlighted in this study, represent the exceptions rather than the norm in presidential health. Courage in facing illness or danger has been characteristic of stricken presidents. The judgment of incapacitated presidents is what often has been lacking.

James Polk

James Polk, the 11th president of the United States, is another example of the resilient nature of the men who have held the office of American president. Polk was never healthy throughout his life. As a child he was small and frail with poor physical endurance. Later in life this was attributed to chronic kidney and bladder infections and the development of a bladder stone. In his early 20s, likely in the year 1816, he traveled 250 miles to consult with a Dr. Ephraim McDowell, a well-renowned surgeon, who diagnosed a urinary bladder stone and recommended surgery.[9]

Brandy was administered as the anesthesia while Polk was held down by assistants and restraining straps. An incision was made in the perineum, the area between the genitals and the anus, and the incision was then extended down through the prostate gland and the wall of the urinary bladder with a gorget, a sharp, chisel-type instrument designed for this purpose. The bladder stone was identified and removed from the bladder with forceps. Remarkably, in an age before sterile surgical fields or antibiotics, Polk survived the surgery without infection, fistula (a remaining open tract between the bladder and the perineal incision) or hemorrhage. Polk married but never had any children. His six married siblings all had families.

Twenty-first century surgery for prostate gland removal, usually performed because of prostate cancer, emphasizes sparing of the nerve bundles adjacent to the prostate gland, which are necessary for subsequent erectile function. Destruction of the nerves guarantees impotence post-operatively. Polk's surgery transected the prostate gland and likely

---

[9] Some biographers of James Polk suggest that his illness was due to gallstones and his surgery a cholecystectomy, removal of the gall bladder. This seems unlikely as the first recorded successful cholecystectomy in this country was in 1867, 50 years after Polk's procedure. Polk's procedure was also described before the Kentucky State Medical Society in 1856 by a Dr. Gross. The description is of a bladder stone removal, not a cholecystectomy.

the adjacent nerves. Although highly progressive for his era and likely life-saving, the surgery probably also rendered him sexually impotent.

Franklin Pierce

Franklin Pierce was the 14th president of the United States. His entrance into politics was preordained. His father was a Revolutionary War hero and twice elected governor of New Hampshire. Young Pierce was elected to the state legislature by age 25 and to the United States Congress by age 29. He also developed a taste for alcohol and an inability to tolerate it as a young man.

Despite his political successes, Pierce led a life filled with tragedy. His wife, who disliked the society and climate of Washington, D.C., suffered two miscarriages and thereafter stayed in New Hampshire during Pierce's congressional years. Pierce lived a "spirited" bachelor's lifestyle with other congressmen. Heavy drinking was a nightly ritual. He battled alcoholism for the remainder of his life.

He retired from Congress and returned to private law practice in New Hampshire in 1842. Living at home and with his wife, his drinking abated. He later served as a general in the Mexican War. Although he did not see combat he shared in the success of the American victory.

At the Democratic Party National Convention of 1852, Pierce became a compromise candidate as the front-runners failed to achieve a majority for nomination. Pierce was nominated on the 49th ballot of that convention. In spite of the fractured Democratic Party, Franklin Pierce was elected the 14th president of the United States.

Shortly before returning to Washington, D.C. to begin his term, the Pierces suffered another tragedy. They were involved in a train derailment accident. Bennie, Pierce's only child, was killed while his parents suffered nary a scratch.

Pierce's term was besieged by the divisions over slavery, pushing the country inevitably toward the Civil War. Congress, with the support of Pierce, gave the Kansas Territory the right to determine its own fate, either slave or free. Zealots from both pro-slavery and abolitionist factions migrated to the Kansas Territory hoping to influence the outcome of the slavery question in Kansas and possibly ultimately in the nation. Consequently, the Kansas Territory became a bloody battleground be-

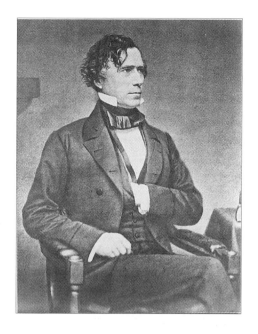

Franklin Pierce, the 14th president of the United States, one of America's most handsome presidents, but also ranked by historians as one of its worst.

tween pro-slavery and abolitionist factions. The Kansas affair irrevocably tarnished Pierce's presidency. He was denied his party's nomination in 1856 for a second term.

After the completion of his term, Pierce returned to New Hampshire, and then toured Europe with his wife. His drinking accelerated upon her death in 1863. Medical biographers believe Pierce's prolonged excess use of alcohol caused alcoholic cirrhosis of the liver.[10] Although he found religion and stopped drinking in 1865, his liver disease progressed and he died in a coma consistent with hepatic coma resulting from liver failure in 1869, a man already forgotten by history.

---

[10] Cirrhosis of the liver is the end stage of alcoholic liver disease. Alcohol is toxic to the liver. A linear correlation generally exists between the dose and duration of alcohol abuse and the development of liver disease. Prolonged use leads progressively to fat deposition in the liver, hepatitis or inflammation and death of liver cells, and cirrhosis or the shrinking and scarring of a severely damaged liver. Ten to 15 percent of heavy drinkers develop cirrhosis of the liver.

CHAPTER 2

Death in the White House

THE UNITED STATES of America was a fragile institution at its inception. With divisions dating to the drafting of the Constitution between the commercial and abolitionist northern states and the agricultural and slave-holding southern states, it was almost as if Lady Luck, Providence (or you may supply your own term) was indeed smiling upon the creation of the United States of America with the health of its early presidents. The struggling republic in its formative years was spared from further divisive issues that may have resulted from presidential disability or death.

William Henry Harrison and John Tyler

Death did not visit the presidency until over 60 years after the formation of the union. William Henry Harrison, "Old Tippecanoe," was elected the ninth president of the United States in 1840. Much like Jackson, Harrison developed his reputation as a military commander. He fought in the Indian wars and the War of 1812. Candidacy of another military hero was not by accident, but an attempt by the Whig Party to counter the popularity of Jackson and his Democratic Party. At the time of the 1840 election, Jackson's Democratic Party had held presidential office for 12 years. Jackson served two terms from 1828-1836, and Martin Van Buren, the vice president in Jackson's second term and Jackson's selection as his successor, fulfilled one term from 1836-1840. The presidential campaign of 1840 was the first truly national campaign with the first campaign slogan, "Tippecanoe and Tyler, Too," referring to Harrison and his vice presidential nominee, John Tyler. The Whigs portrayed Harrison as a log-cabin-born, frontier-raised and hard-cider-drinking common man. In other words, he was portrayed to be more Jacksonian than Jackson, and it worked.

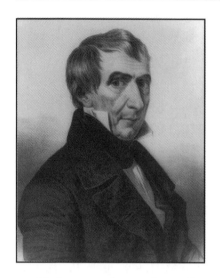

William Henry Harrison, the ninth president of the United States. Courtesy of Library of Congress Prints and Photographs.

But somewhere along the way it may have been forgotten that Harrison was an old man, 68 years old when he assumed the presidency, the oldest man to assume the presidency until Ronald Reagan a century and a half later.

Harrison sank immediately underneath his presidential burden. Harrison's inauguration occurred on March 4, 1841, in Washington, D.C. The weather was cold and blustery, not unusual for Washington, D.C. in March. Harrison delivered the longest inaugural address on record, pontificating for one hour and 40 minutes, wearing neither coat nor hat. He immediately became ill and could not attend the receptions in his honor that evening.

After assuming office, Harrison was besieged by spoil seekers. During the campaign, either because his memory failed or as a strategy to gather support, Harrison had promised the same government positions to two or three different individuals. The resulting chaos over patronage further sapped his strength.

Three weeks after taking office he came down with pneumonia, a serious, often fatal disease in that time. His medical treatment, however, did not help. Medical theory of the day maintained that illness was caused by bad "humors" trapped in the body. Treatment involved permitting those humors to escape the body. Remedies usually involved elimination of body fluids, hopefully with the accompanying evil humors. Accepted therapies included blood letting, usually accomplished by cutting or lancing the antecubital vein in the bend of the elbow. Cupping was a less invasive form of blood letting in which an area of the skin was scratched and a heated glass cup inverted and applied to the scarified skin. As the cup cooled, a vacuum formed drawing blood and fluids to the skin surface. Finally, emetics and cathartics were used to dispel fluids and humors through the bowel by inducing vomiting or bowel movements respectively.

Harrison received all of these treatments at various times during his illness. He also was given calomel, brandy, laudanum, castor oil and opium as medicines.[11] Not surprisingly, this 68-year-old man got worse. His fever increased. He developed gastrointestinal symptoms and jaundice. On April 4, 1841, exactly one month after his inauguration, William Henry Harrison became the first president to die in office. Of all American presidents, he had by far the shortest tenure in office. Historians give his presidency an incomplete grade. Although his illness would almost certainly be curable by 21st century medicine, his brief presidential occupancy offers no clues as to how history may have differed or been impacted had he lived to serve out his elected term.

Probably the most historical aspect of Harrison's death was the ultimate effect on the office of vice president. The vice president's role in government was quite limited in those times. Vice President John Tyler was living on his Virginia plantation and did not even know that Harrison was ill. Upon Harrison's death, a rider was dispatched from Washington, D.C. to inform Tyler of Harrison's passing. Tyler was a southerner from Virginia. He was a former Democrat and relatively recent convert to the Whig Party at the time of his nomination. He had been added to the Whig Party ticket for geographic and political balance.

The Constitution was vague on exactly what the duties of the vice

---

[11] Laudanum was an opium-based painkiller prescribed for multiple illnesses and also used as a recreational drug in the 18th century. The drug was obtained from poppies and then mixed with sugar and/or alcohol to make it easier to drink. Calomel was a mercury compound (mercurous chloride) prescribed to clear the intestines, stimulate the liver, and otherwise help heal the body. Oral ulcers often occurred with moderate use, and mercury poisoning causing multiple systemic symptoms could result with repetitive, heavy use.

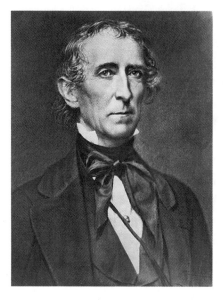

John Tyler, the 10th president of the United States and the first vice president to assume office after the death of a president. Courtesy of Library of Congress Prints and Photographs.

president were upon the death of the elected president. The wording is as follows:

"In Case of the removal of the President from **Office,** *or of his Death, Resignation, or Inability to discharge* **the Powers and Duties** *of the said Office, the Same shall devolve on the Vice President..."* (bolding added for emphasis by the author).

Some believed that the **duties** became those of the vice president but **not** the **office** itself, and that the vice president was only the acting president. Even Tyler's cabinet, which he inherited from Harrison, wanted decisions to be made by committee with Tyler having an equal but not overriding vote.

Tyler, an Icabod Crane look-alike, was referred to as "His Accidency." He received letters addressed to him as either the Vice President or the Acting President, letters which he returned unopened with "address unknown" written on the envelope. Tyler claimed and discharged the full authority of the office of president of the United States, thus setting the precedent for all future vice presidents ascending to office on the death of a president. Tyler made liberal use of the presidential veto. Unfortunately, his views often conflicted with the members of his cabinet and his own party. All but one of his cabinet members resigned during his term. Tyler, the sitting although unelected president, was expelled from his own political party during his single term in office. He retired after completing the elected term of Harrison and returned to Virginia.

At the outset of the Civil War, Tyler was elected to the Congress of the Confederacy. He traveled to Richmond, Virginia, the capital of the Confederacy, but died of an apparent stroke just prior to assuming this post. His gravesite was ignored by the United States government for over a century after his death, but his legacy remains intact. John Tyler clearly established that the vice president is indeed only a heartbeat away from the presidency.[12]

Zachary Taylor

Less than 10 years later a similar situation transpired in the history of presidential health. Zachary Taylor was elected the 12th president of the United States and assumed office in 1849. The Whig Party again chose a military hero as their candidate, following a political formula first successful for Andrew Jackson and then for William Henry Harrison. Taylor was elected largely on his popularity as a victorious general in several battles of the Mexican War. In dispute was the Mexican/American border. The war resulted in the addition of lands to the United States which now comprise parts of the states of California, Arizona, New Mexico and Texas. "Old Rough and Ready" was a career Army officer who centered his campaign on this popularity rather than policy or strong party affiliation. He stated, "If elected, I would not be the mere president of a party — I would endeavor to act independent of party domina-

---

[12] The office of vice president remained vacant during the remainder of Tyler's presidency. There was no mechanism outlined by the Constitution for selection of a vice president, if and when a former vice president assumed the presidency. Tyler had a brush with death late in his presidency. A large presidential party boarded a new steam-powered battleship, the USS Princeton, for a cruise on the Potomac River. The highlight of the cruise was the firing of the ship's new cannons. The guns were fired spectacularly and uneventfully several times, but upon the last firing, one of the cannons exploded, killing several on deck instantly, including two members of Tyler's cabinet. Tyler was safely below deck when the explosion occurred. If the Constitution was vague on succession on death of the president, it was silent on the death of both the president and vice president during the term of office. One can only imagine the chaos that may have erupted if Tyler had been killed on that fateful day.

tion, and should feel bound to administer the government untrammeled by party schemes ..."

Taylor, like Harrison, was not a young man. He was 64 years old when he took the oath of office and 65 years old at the time of his death. Taylor first became ill on July 4, 1850. On this typical, hot, muggy, Washington, D.C. summer day, Taylor attended a celebration at the Washington Monument. He then took a long walk before returning to the White House. By the time he reached the White House, he was hungry and thirsty. He consumed a large quantity of raw fruit, reportedly apples and cherries. He also drank large quantities of iced water and milk. Remember, this was a time before pasteurization, water purification or protections against food contamination. At dinner that evening he again indulged in cold liquids and cherries. His physician, Dr. Watherspoon, who happened to dine with President Taylor that evening, admonished the president for his overindulgences and his poor dietary habits.

The doctor's warnings were prophetic, but too late. Later that evening Taylor developed abdominal discomfort with nausea and cramps. This progressed to diarrhea, vomiting and fever. Dr. Watherspoon's diagnosis was cholera morbus, a general diagnosis covering almost any gastrointestinal illnesses.

The description of Taylor's symptoms could be consistent with gastroenteritis, cholecystitis, diverticulitis, pancreatitis, etc.[13] Whatever the acute gastrointestinal ailment was, it proved fatal in the 19th century and would likely be treatable and curable today. Once again a president was subjected to blood letting in attempts at a cure. President Taylor

---

13 Gastroenteritis is a syndrome characterized by vomiting, watery diarrhea and abdominal cramps. It can be caused by one of several viruses. Usually it tends to be self-limited, but more persistent cases can occur due to bacterial infection or food poisoning. Cholecystitis is inflammation of the gallbladder wall, usually caused by a gallstones obstructing normal flow of bile from the gall bladder to the small bowel. After stabilization, surgical removal of the gall bladder, now usually done by a laproscopic technique, is usually curative. Diverticulitis is inflammation of diverticulae, sac-like out-pouchings of the wall of the large bowel. If an inflamed diverticula perforates allowing the bacteria normally in the bowel access to the abdominal cavity, abscess (a local pocket of bacterial infection) or peritonitis (generalized intra-abdominal infection) can result.

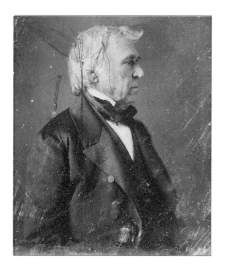

Profile of Zachary Taylor, the 12th president of the United States. Courtesy of Library of Congress Prints and Photographs.

died on July 9, four days after his dietary indiscretion and after serving just over one year in office.

With almost every American presidential death in office there has been an accompanying conspiracy theory. Such was the case with President Zachary Taylor.

Theorists speculated that Taylor's death may not have been natural, but related to poisoning by individuals angered by Taylor's political views.[14] In this case, the voices of the conspiracy theorists became stri-

---

[14] Zachary Taylor was a political neophyte. He had never held office or even voted prior to the election of 1848 when he became president. Taylor's selection as president hinged upon his reputation as a military hero. He did not embrace any platform or issues as a candidate. Taylor was a southerner by birth, a slave owner, and was elected with significant support from the southern states. However, as president he opposed the expansion of slavery to new states or territories. He was committed to the Union at all costs and rejected the concept of a state's right of secession from the Union. His views were actually quite similar to another American president a decade later, Abraham Lincoln. Taylor opposed the Compromise of 1850, a multifaceted bill with the following provisions:
- California admitted to Union as a state free of slavery
- Borders of Texas defined
- Territories of New Mexico and Utah established with self determination by residents whether those territories would allow or prohibit slavery.
- The Fugitive Slave Act which required federal government to actively return runaway slaves to their owners. Suspected fugitives had no right to trial or judicial proceeding. Therefore, legally free blacks, if claimed, could be *(cont. next page)*

dent enough that the body of Zachary Taylor was exhumed from its crypt in Zachary Taylor National Cemetery in Louisville, Kentucky, in 1991. Tissue samples were removed and examined by NMR (nuclear magnetic resonance) techniques. No evidence of poisoning was found. Hopefully, now the conspiracy theorists as well as President Taylor can rest in peace.

Warren G. Harding

Until John F. Kennedy's assassination, no president's death generated more suspicion than that of Warren G. Harding. He died suddenly and unexpectedly, at least to the American public, at age 57, just as details of personal indiscretions and administrative scandals emerged. Harding, the 29th president of the United States, assumed office in 1921. Prior to that he was a senator from Ohio, who in his six-year term authored no major pieces of legislation and missed two-thirds of the roll call votes. Still, in 1920 the deadlocked Republican Party National Convention nominated the affable, if undistinguished, Harding.

As one historian put it, "He was probably the least qualified candidate ever nominated by a major party." Even by his own admission, Harding was overmatched by the job. He stated as president, "I listen to one side and they seem right, and then — God! — I talk to the other side and they seem just as right, and here I am where I started. I know somewhere there is a book that will give me the truth, but hell! I couldn't read the book."

His administration was a disaster, the most corrupt administration in American history. Several scandals occurred during Harding's brief

---

and were returned to their presumed owners without due process. Heavy criminal and civil penalties were established for citizens aiding fugitive slaves.

Taylor planned to veto the bill if passed by Congress. Lack of this compromise may have led to secession of Texas or South Carolina and a test of Union forces versus the seceded state's troops on a more limited scale than the eventual Civil War. Millard Fillmore, Taylor's successor, supported the bill which eventually became law. This compromise temporarily avoided civil unrest but the implementation of the Fugitive Slave Act hardened both northern and southern positions and was one of many steps which ultimately led to the Civil War.

tenure.[15] Harding himself, although unknown at the time, continued to have extramarital affairs.[16]

Harding first experienced angina[17] in 1922. In January of 1923

---

[15] In the Teapot Dome scandal Harding's secretary of the interior leased government oil reserves in Wyoming and California to private developers and received payments for doing so. Elsewhere, officials of the Veteran's Bureau awarded contracts based on who offered the biggest kickback. One Veteran's Bureau official committed suicide when the Bureau's transgressions became public. Officials in the attorney general's office arranged protection from raids by prohibition agents to those involved in bootlegging. (The 18th Amendment established prohibition of alcoholic beverages in 1920. The 21st Amendment repealed Prohibition in 1933.) Another suicide occurred as a result of this scandal. The attorney general was aware of the graft but did nothing.

[16] Secret love letters between Harding and Carrie Fulton Phillips, the wife of a longtime friend of Harding, were released in 1963. The letters revealed an intermittent 15-year love affair. Mrs. Phillips unsuccessfully pressured Harding to leave his wife. She moved to Germany, and later returned to America as an outspoken German advocate. She threatened to reveal Harding's tryst with her unless Harding, now a senator, voted against the declaration of war with Germany in World War I. Harding voted in favor of the resolution, and Mrs. Phillips abandoned her threat. The affair continued until Harding won the Republican presidential nomination in 1920. To avoid a scandal during the campaign, the Republican National Committee bribed the Phillips for their cooperation with a cash payment, a monthly stipend, and a slow cruise to Japan.

Harding had a second affair with Nan Britton, a lady 30 years younger than Harding, which began in 1917. According to Ms. Britton's account, she conceived a child born in 1919, and Harding paid generous child support, with payments often hand-delivered by Secret Service agents. Trysts continued through Harding's Senate and White House years. After the death of Mr. and Mrs. Harding, Britton lobbied unsuccessfully for a trust fund for her daughter from the Harding estate. Rebuffed, she wrote a scandalous book, *The President's Daughter* (1927), dedicated to "all unwed mothers." It became a best seller.

[17] Angina is characterized by precordial (mid-chest) pressure or discomfort, typically brought on by exertion or emotion and relieved by rest. The cause is usually critical coronary artery obstruction due to atherosclerosis. The coronary arteries carry blood and nutrients to the heart muscle. Symptoms occur when the energy needs of the heart muscle exceed the capacity of the arteries obstructed by atherosclerosis to supply these needs. Individuals with angina are at risk of myocardial infarction (heart attack), permanent damage to the heart muscle caused by total occlusion of a coronary vessel and cessation of blood flow to an area of the heart.

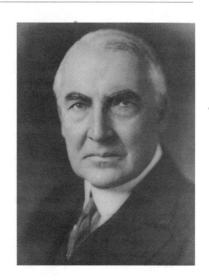

Warren G. Harding, the 29th president of the United States, won the nomination of the Republican Party and then the general election in 1920. Courtesy of Library of Congress Prints and Photo-

Harding suffered an attack of "flu" which, in retrospect, was likely a myocardial infarction (heart attack) that precipitated a rapidly downward course. Harding had at least two currently recognized risk factors for heart disease. He had high blood pressure and he was a smoker. In fact, Harding enjoyed tobacco in all forms, smoking cigars, a pipe and occasional cigarettes. He also chewed tobacco. Thomas Edison endorsed the president's habits, once stating, "Any man who chews tobacco is all right." Harding also had central obesity, weight accumulation primarily around the waist, which has recently also been associated with an increased risk of diabetes and cardiovascular diseases.

The public was not aware of any problems. This may be in large part because the president's personal physician, a Dr. Charles Sawyer, never suspected heart disease.

Dr. Sawyer was an interesting choice as Harding's personal physician. He was a homeopathic physician. He first became acquainted with the Harding family through Harding's parents, both of whom were also homeopathic physicians. Homeopathy was a small branch of medicine based on two principles:

- The law of *similia,* which states that a disease state will be cured by medications that produce the same symptoms in a healthy person as exhibited by the illness.
- The law of infinitesimals, which states that the smaller a dose of medicine given, the more effective the treatment is in healing. Put

another way, the more minute a drug dosage, the more potent its curative potential.

Consequently, homeopathic physicians tended to be minimalists in their approach to disease. Although the laws of homeopathy have largely been refuted, the relative non-invasive approach of homeopathic physicians may have been superior to the techniques such as bleeding, cathartics and emetics employed by main-line physicians of the 19th century.

Much acrimony existed between the allopathic or mainline physicians and homeopathic physicians in the 19th century, but by the 20th century relations between the different medical branches had improved, and Sawyer's appointment as the president's physician caused little controversy.

Sawyer never diagnosed heart disease. That something was wrong was obvious to others. Dr. Emmanuel Libman, a physician specializing in heart diseases, encountered Harding at a Washington, D.C. dinner party in the fall of 1922. After observing the president's color, obesity and shortness of breath, he opined to a friend that, "The president has a disease of the coronary arteries." He predicted the president would be dead within six months. Even the White House valet, Arthur Brooks, sensed trouble. He confided to a Secret Service agent in early 1923, "… something is going to happen to our boss. He can't sleep at night. He can't lie down. He has to be propped up on pillows, and he sits up that way all night. If he lies down, he can't get his breath." The valet described classic symptoms of congestive heart failure.[18] Harding's congestive heart failure was not medically recognized or treated at that time.

[18] Congestive heart failure is dysfunction of the heart muscle leading to fluid overload, accumulation of fluid in the lungs, internal organs (especially the liver) and peripheral tissues (especially the lower extremities). Symptoms are shortness of breath with activity, shortness of breath when lying flat and edema. Systolic heart failure refers to dysfunction of the pumping action of the heart muscle. Diseases such as heart attacks due to coronary artery disease, hypertension, severe narrowing or leakage of the heart valves can all lead to systolic heart muscle dysfunction. More recently recognized is the importance of the diastolic properties of the heart muscle, i.e., the ability of the heart muscle to relax, expand and accept blood flow from the lungs during the period of time between heartbeats. With diastolic dysfunction, the heart becomes more rigid, less distensible and requires *(cont. next page)*

President Harding scheduled a cruise to Alaska to dedicate the Alaska Railroad by driving the final golden spike into place. With some reservation, Dr. Sawyer agreed. Although concerned about the rigors of a transcontinental railroad trip, the stresses of remaining in Washington, D.C. during the escalating Senate investigation into the Harding administration were also potentially daunting.

Harding's health deteriorated on the cross-country trek. During a stop in Vancouver, Canada, on the return trip, he could not complete a round of golf. He was transferred from the front nine to the final hole so he could appear to finish and not raise suspicions of his failing health. During a later stop in Seattle he nearly collapsed while delivering a speech. Harding was then swiftly transported by rail to San Francisco, where he was placed at bed rest at the Palace Hotel. Leading heart doctors were summoned to examine Harding and consult with Dr. Sawyer.

Although it seems curious Harding was placed in a hotel rather than a hospital, hospitals, when established in the late 1700s, were facilities for care of the impoverished, insane and terminally ill rather than a place for treatment or cure. This perception lingered into the early 20th century.

Harding was diagnosed with an enlarged heart, bronchial pneumonia and, finally, congestive heart failure. He did not receive an electrocardiogram.[19]

---

higher vascular pressures to fill the pumping chamber in preparation for the next heart beat. These elevated pressures are transmitted to the lungs, causing the fluid retention and the symptoms of heart failure above. The diseases that cause diastolic abnormalities of the heart muscle are similar to those that cause systolic dysfunction. Many patients with symptomatic congestive heart failure probably have elements of both systolic and diastolic myocardial dysfunction contributing to their symptoms.

[19] The electrocardiogram, a recording from the chest wall of the electrical activity of the heart, was developed by William Einthoven in Germany in 1901. The original equipment to record an electrocardiogram weighed nearly 600 pounds, took up two rooms and required five people to operate. It became available to the medical community in parts of America by 1910. The characteristic changes that occur in the electrocardiogram during a myocardial infarction were described by Herrick in 1918. Whether this knowledge and a *portable* electrocardiogram were available to the San Francisco physicians in 1923 is highly problematic. The electrocardiogram remains an important test in detecting heart attack today.

He apparently did receive digitalis,[20] which suggests Dr. Sawyer consented to the suggestions of the orthodox physicians gathered.

Two days later Harding was resting and listening to his wife read an article favorable to the president. Harding remarked, "That's good, read some more." These were his last words. Shortly thereafter, his body suddenly slumped. His mouth fell open and he became unresponsive. His physicians were nearby but could not revive him.

Interestingly, the physicians, apparently deferring to Dr. Sawyer's judgment, listed the cause of death as "apoplexy," lexicon of the day for a stroke. Clearly, with angina, a probable myocardial infarction, an enlarged heart, congestive heart failure and the description of his demise, Harding died of sudden cardiac death, likely due to a ventricular arrhythmia.[21]

Mrs. Harding refused an autopsy. Rumors later arose of foul play causing Harding's death, but there is no historical evidence to support these speculations.

Harding's death from complications of undiagnosed and untreated coronary artery disease 80 years ago adds perspective to the remarkable

---

[20] Digitalis, an herbal medication first identified in the 1700s in England, is created from dried powdered leaf of the flowering plant foxglove (digitalis purpurea). Digitalis exerts its action by increasing the strength of contraction of failing heart muscle. Synthetic medications based on digitalis are still in use today for heart failure and irregular heart rhythms.

[21] Under normal conditions specialized electrical cells in the atria (collecting chambers) of the heart act as the pacemaker of the heart, establish the heart's rhythm and rate, and promote coordinated heart muscle contraction. However, with either weakness of the heart muscle or ischemia, lack of blood supply to the heart, the muscle cells of the ventricles become electrically irritable and may usurp the pacemaker duties of the heart by establishing a faster heart rate (ventricular tachycardia). When this occurs, coordinated pumping of the heart is lost and blood pressure and output of blood from the heart may fall. Also, ventricular tachycardia is an unstable rhythm which often deteriorates further into chaotic electrical activity with no effective contraction of the heart (ventricular fibrillation). Unless corrected by defibrillation, an electrical shock either applied externally to the chest or internally by a previously placed automatic implantable defibrillator, this is a fatal heart rhythm and rapidly causes death. Up to 50 percent of deaths due to heart disease ultimately occur from sudden death due to a ventricular arrhythmia *(see footnote 43)*.

gains in the treatment of coronary artery disease over a relatively short period of time. Today options in his care would include antihypertensive and cholesterol-lowering medications to lower heart attack risk. When symptoms developed, then coronary artery angiograms would be performed to determine if coronary angioplasty, coronary artery stents or coronary artery bypass surgery might be beneficial. Automatic implantable defibrillators to detect and treat life-threatening heart rhythms, which likely claimed Harding's life, and electrical bi-ventricular pacemakers which reduce the symptoms of heart failure, may have been employed and beneficial.

As reports of administrative corruption and personal improprieties became public, Harding became somewhat of a national joke, and then, forgotten by history. Harding is consistently ranked last in surveys of historians grading presidential administrations.

Had he lived, Harding faced impeachment and/or conviction by Congress for the scandals of his administration and either resignation or eviction from office. It is sad but true that death in office was, historically, the most satisfactory outcome for Harding's presidency.

Franklin Delano Roosevelt

Franklin Delano Roosevelt was the 32nd president of the United States and the only president elected to more than two terms. In his 12-plus years in office, Roosevelt aroused a loyalty and opposition unequaled in American history. But as the architect of the New Deal, the Great Society, and the president who led the country out of the Great Depression and on to victory in World War II, even critics must view him among America's great presidents. But Roosevelt was never forthcoming regarding his health and disability.

In 1920, 12 years before becoming president, Roosevelt was paralyzed in the lower extremities by an attack of polio.[22] Roosevelt re-

22 Polio is an acute viral infection caused by the polio virus. The disease is highly contagious and several major epidemics of polio have occurred in the United States. Most cases are self-limited, but the virus can attack the central nervous system and lead to paralysis, especially in children. President Roosevelt announced the creation of the National Foundation for Infantile Paralysis in 1938, a campaign to combat polio which became recognized by the slogan, "March of Dimes." It seemed

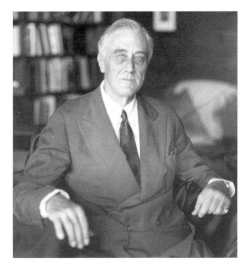

The last photographic portrait of Franklin Delano Roosevelt, the 32nd president of the United States, taken in 1945, only days before his death in Warm Springs, Georgia. Courtesy of Library of Congress Prints and Photographs.

quired heavy metal leg braces and assistance to walk. He spent the majority of his time in a wheelchair, but of the over 5,000 pictures available during his White House years, only two show him in a wheelchair.

He, with assistance from his staff, became adept at swinging his legs out of the car and locking his braces simultaneously to give the appearance of mobility. The vast majority of Americans did not realize their president was physically disabled. Although this continued a disturbing pattern of the American presidency, i.e., secrecy and privacy in matters of health, this was not limiting to Roosevelt's completion of his presidential duties. (Hidden illnesses in the White House are further explored in the third chapter.)

Roosevelt selected Admiral Ross McIntire as his personal physician at the outset of his White House years. McIntire was recommended to Roosevelt by Admiral Cary Grayson, who was Woodrow Wilson's personal physician. (See Chapter 3 for additional information on Grayson's serendipitous appointment.) Dr. McIntire was an ear, nose and throat specialist. His major treatments of Roosevelt over the years consisted of nasal drops and sinus irrigations for Roosevelt's frequent upper respira-

natural after his death to honor Roosevelt by placing his portrait on a new dime coin. This was done in 1946. Vaccines, first the Salk vaccine in 1955 and later the oral Sabin vaccine in 1962, have essentially eliminated the disease of polio in civilized countries.

tory infections and symptoms. Indeed, the nasal drops may have worsened Roosevelt's hypertension.

However, in late 1943 Roosevelt's health became a major concern. He had recurrent headaches, cough, general malaise and fatigue. First, his symptoms were ascribed to the flu, then post-flu syndrome, then bronchitis by Dr. McIntire. McIntire's position regarding Roosevelt's health, which he maintained up to Roosevelt's death, was that Roosevelt was in the best of health for a man of his age. But Roosevelt's symptoms persisted, even worsened over the next six months. In March of 1944 at the insistence of Roosevelt's daughter, a second opinion was obtained from a cardiologist, Dr. Bruenn. His findings and treatment may have extended Roosevelt's life.

Dr. Bruenn discovered a blood pressure of 180/110 mmHg (normal 120/80 mm Hg), an enlarged heart, lung congestion, and leakage of the mitral valve. He correctly diagnosed congestive heart failure (see Footnote 18). hypertension, hypertensive cardiovascular disease (heart failure related to long-standing hypertension) and, possibly to appease Dr. McIntire, acute bronchitis. Roosevelt was started on digitalis (see footnote 20) with significant improvement in heart failure symptoms but no improvement in his blood pressure, which actually worsened, increasing to the 200-240 mmHg systolic and 110-120 mmHg diastolic range.

The problem is that even with treatment, Dr. Bruenn's diagnosis was a fatal one in 1944. Although there were limited treatments for congestive heart failure, there were no effective pharmacologic treatments for hypertension. Severe hypertension was the primary cause of Roosevelt's physical predicament. Roosevelt had incipient malignant hypertension, the end stage of hypertension, which invariably leads to heart failure, kidney failure, neurologic events or any combination of the above. The diagnosis of malignant hypertension conveyed a life expectancy of about one year.

Roosevelt's health was not released to the public. In fact, there is evidence that Roosevelt himself did not know or particularly care to inquire about the status of his health. Dr. Bruenn, a reserve naval officer, was instructed to report exclusively to Dr. McIntire and not report findings or treatments to the patient, Roosevelt. Interestingly, Bruenn later observed that Roosevelt had a strange ambivalence regarding his health. Roosevelt never inquired about his blood pressure, his medications or even what type of doctor the good Dr. Bruenn was. Whether this was a denial mechanism or an historic struggle to complete his presidential responsibilities remains unknown.

Those responsibilities demanded Roosevelt's attention to substantial domestic and international issues. In 1944 World War II was in progress. Preparations for military assaults into Europe and the Far East were proceeding. Domestically, it was an election year. Roosevelt, relying on the Lincoln wartime dictum established during the Civil War, "… it is best not to change horses in the middle of a stream," ignored his health and decided to run for re-election. Roosevelt's nomination was assured by his candidacy, but whispers and rumors of his failing health emerged at the Democratic Party National Convention. Many viewed the selection of Roosevelt's running mate tantamount to election of the next president. Henry Wallace, vice president during Roosevelt's third term, was considered a left-winger by many in his own Democratic Party. He was dumped from the ticket in favor of a former haberdasher turned senator from Missouri, Harry Truman.

The press of that era printed only the most favorable photographs of Roosevelt. An editor of the magazine *Life* later opined, "We decided to print the ones that were least bad and – by trying to lean over backwards to be fair — we infringed our contract with the readers to tell the truth — that Roosevelt was a dying man,"

Roosevelt did not attend the Democratic National Convention. He did not campaign until the last three weekends before the election. In an era before television, the American public believed the campaign posters showing a robust Roosevelt. The suppressed photographs of the president showed a marked deterioration and frailty over the last year. Roosevelt won re-election handily.

Roosevelt lost approximately 30 pounds in 1944, the first 10 prescribed by his physician, but the next 20 likely due to cardiac cachexia (generalized muscle-wasting due to his heart failure). His fourth inaugural address, delivered at the White House, was the shortest on record, only a few dozen words. Mrs. Woodrow Wilson, widow of Woodrow Wilson *(see Chapter 3),* was a guest that day at the White House. On seeing the president, she prophetically observed, "He looks exactly as my husband did when he went into his decline."

Shortly after the inauguration Roosevelt traveled 14,000 miles to Yalta to meet with Churchill and Stalin for negotiations on the make-up of post-war Europe. Clearly, America was represented by an impaired president. Churchill's physician told associates that the president had "all the symptoms of hardening of the arteries of the brain ... so I give him a few months to live." The White House screened all photographs taken of the president and, with an accommodating press, suppressed the worst and only allowed the kindest to appear in print. Even these told the story of a dying president. Still, by most accounts, Roosevelt remained effective at the Yalta conference. Future failure of that accord can be ascribed to the USSR's non-compliance.[23]

Roosevelt returned to America and Warm Springs, Georgia, his little White House. There the inevitable occurred. While sitting for a portrait on April 12, 1945, he developed a sudden, severe headache and quickly collapsed into unconsciousness. Dr. Bruenn was nearby and quickly attended the president. Bruenn's examination showed a comatose patient with a rigid neck, a dilated right pupil and systolic blood pressure over 300 mm Hg. The president had suffered a massive cerebral hemorrhage (bleeding into the brain due to rupture of a blood vessel). He died within two hours.[24] He survived only three months of his elected four-year

---

[23] The Yalta Conference began in February 1945, a time when victory in Europe was all but assured, but during continuing conflict with Japan. Yalta, a city on the Black Sea in Crimea, was a location of Stalin's choosing and clearly on his turf. One objective for the United States was to coax Stalin and the USSR to join the war against Japan after Germany's imminent surrender, a goal less valuable in retrospect considering the development of the atomic bomb. A second goal was to equitably determine post-war occupation and governance of Germany and Poland. The Red Army already occupied most of Poland and eastern Europe, and consequently these areas were likely outside any influence from Roosevelt or Churchill. Hopes to restore the previous Polish government rather than a communistic regime chosen by Stalin proved futile. In the division of Germany, the Allied Forces acquired control over the industrial heartland versus the largely agricultural eastern regions that fell to Soviet authority.

[24] The brain surrounded by the inflexible skull (cranium) is in an enclosed space. Bleeding into the brain becomes life-threatening because of a rise in intracranial pressure which squeezes the brain tissue and causes dysfunction. The midbrain,

term. No autopsy was done, but atherosclerosis was so severe that the undertakers had difficulty embalming the body.

As one columnist for the *Saturday Evening Post* opined, "The state of Mr. Roosevelt's health was a secret from millions of Americans who voted for the president on the theory that he could reasonably be expected to live out his term in office, where he was indispensable if America was to achieve a strong and lasting peace." Americans had unwittingly placed their trust for a just peace on the shoulders of a dying man.

So the country was forced to "change horses." Roosevelt had not prepped Truman of any military, diplomatic or administrative matters save for a casual reference to the atomic bomb. It was a portrait for disaster. Fortunately, Truman surpassed expectations as president. Historians generally praise Truman's management of the conclusion of World War II, including use of the atomic bomb in Japan to shorten the Asian conflict.

---

where the involuntary centers for consciousness and breathing reside, is forced downward into the bony opening at the base of the skull. Resulting midbrain dysfunction leads to unconsciousness and death.

CHAPTER 3

Hidden Illnesses in the White House

TO ME, THE most intriguing aspect of presidential health is how presidents, their administrations and their physicians have responded to presidential illnesses. Presidential illness creates a conflict. Presidents, like all individuals, have a right to privacy in medical matters. But the public has the right to know any circumstances which might impact the effectiveness of its elected leaders. Presidential physicians can be ethically ensnared between a duty to their presidential patient and a separate duty to maintain the public trust. Other administrative officials face the same dilemma. Practically, responsibility to the chief executive has trumped duty to the public in almost all instances where the conflict has occurred. Maybe this is not surprising considering that the basis of all administrative positions is the president. All appointees serve at the discretion of the president. Their station and whatever power and influence that station entails originates with the president. If the president becomes disabled, their office and power may become impotent or non-existent. Therefore, there is a major disinclination of administrative officials, and this extends additionally to family members as well, to identify presidential limitations, whether health or otherwise. Still, historically it is compelling the lengths to which presidents, administrative officials, physicians and family members have gone to conceal presidential illness.

The American media and presidential coverage have changed dramatically over the course of the American presidency, especially in the last 50 years with the advent of television. While 19th century political editorials could be widely partisan, presidential coverage was milder and even deferential to the office. Even negative reports were confined to regional rather than national newspapers and print media, sources that never reached the majority of the American citizenry. Currently, the media inundates the populace with political coverage. The media not only reports, but investigates, editorializes and speculates, and ultimately shapes public opinion.

This chapter explores cover-ups of presidential illnesses. A subsequent chapter examines how the media has changed the dynamics of disclosure of such illnesses.

Grover Cleveland

The earliest and possibly most ingenious cover-up of a presidential medical issue involved President Grover Cleveland in 1893. He clandestinely underwent general anesthesia and oral cancer surgery aboard a private yacht steaming up Long Island Sound to Cleveland's summer home in Massachusetts. When rumors of the surgery and the president's illness arose, the White House vigorously denied the story. In other words, Cleveland's administration lied. The full story did not become known until 24 years later when one of the surgeons released his memoirs.

But let's set the stage. Cleveland, the only president elected to non-consecutive terms, was both the 22nd and 24th presidents of the United States. In 1893, during his second term, Cleveland noticed a persistent roughened area on the roof of his mouth. Cleveland, like Grant (see Chapter 7), smoked cigars. After six weeks without improvement, Cleveland sought the counsel of White House physician, Dr. Robert O'Reilly. Initial examination by Dr. O'Reilly showed an ulcer the size of a quarter on the roof of Cleveland's mouth. O'Reilly requested a consultation from Dr. Joseph Bryant, a prominent surgeon. A biopsy specimen was secretly obtained and examined at Johns Hopkins University. The pathologic diagnosis was oral cancer, and immediate surgery was recommended. President Cleveland believed that any signs of weakness or personal illness would doom his plans to return the country to a gold-backed currency.[25] He therefore agreed to surgery, but only if the process was kept absolutely secret.

---

[25] The Sherman Silver Purchase Act, which became law in 1890, effectively established both silver and gold as the precious metals stored in government coffers to guarantee the value of government-issued currency. A bi-metal-backed currency tended to lead to cheaper money and favored borrowers, farmers and especially Western mining interests. However, as mining output of silver rose and silver prices fell,

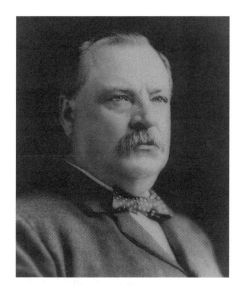

Grover Cleveland, the only man ever elected to non-consecutive terms, was the 22nd and 24th presidents of the United States. Courtesy of Library of Congress Prints and Photographs.

Hasty arrangements were made for clandestine surgery. Cleveland called a special session of Congress to consider repeal of the Sherman Silver Purchase Act for August, six weeks away, to allow time for his surgical recuperation. He then ostentatiously traveled to New York and boarded the *Oneida*, a friend's private yacht which was anchored in New York Harbor. By public accounts President Cleveland was scheduled for a leisure cruise to his home state of Massachusetts, there to enjoy a prolonged summer vacation. However, Cleveland was met secretly on board the yacht by a team of doctors and dentists to perform the surgery. Cleveland's secretary of war was the only administrative official present and also the only cabinet secretary even aware of the planned surgery.

The next morning the ship weighed anchor and proceeded at half-speed up the East River. Bear in mind that President Cleveland was not a svelte specimen. In fact, he was quite obese, over 250 pounds. He was a poor risk for anesthesia, let alone the rigors of the necessary surgery. The doctors prepared the president for surgery by propping him in a

---

more notes were redeemed for the more stable metal, gold. By 1893 federal gold reserves were depleted, and foreign country investments in America declined. Several bankruptcies occurred and a financial panic loomed. Cleveland favored return to a gold standard as a way to stabilize the currency and avoid further financial panic.

chair secured to the interior mast of the ship. Dr. Bryant, lead surgeon, told the captain with obvious anxiety, "If you hit a rock, hit it good and hard so we all go to the bottom."

Nitrous oxide (laughing gas), ether and cocaine were used for anesthesia. All incisions were made inside the mouth. Therefore, if all went well, there would be no outward signs of surgery after the initial bruising and swelling subsided. After the dentist removed two of Cleveland's left front teeth, Dr. Bryant attacked the cancer with an incision in the roof of Cleveland's mouth. The cancer proved to be a gelatinous mass which extended through the bone of the palate (roof of the mouth) into the maxillary sinus (the bony cavity above the mouth but below the nose). To completely excise the tumor, much of the hard palate and parts of the upper jaw bone were removed, painstakingly chiseled away in small pieces. Bleeding was controlled by direct pressure, cold water compresses and primitive electrical cauterization. The operation lasted just under an hour.

It is mystifying why the medical team, composed of five respected physicians and surgeons, consented to the secret surgery. Even in a day before medical malpractice and plaintiff's attorneys, the physicians shouldered enormous personal and professional risk by undertaking the surgery. Certainly, the potential for catastrophe existed. Cleveland was a morbidly obese subject administered volatile and flammable anesthesia, i.e., ether. Primitive electrical equipment for cautery was used which could have ignited the anesthetic gases. Further, a yacht at the mercy of the rising and falling seas did not provide the most stable surgical theater. If Cleveland had not survived the surgery or suffered complications, the surgical team's professional reputations could not have survived. Although one might be able to justify the secretive nature of the surgery as at the request of the patient, performing the surgery unnecessarily under the suboptimal conditions of a ship at sea seems an undefendable medical decision.

Against all odds, the surgery came off without a hitch. Cleveland not only survived, but had no complications. When the presidential entourage disembarked in Massachusetts, the press was informed the president had undergone a tooth extraction. When rumors of more serious surgery arose, further fabrications were concocted by Cleveland's administration. Their explanations appeased the media of Cleveland's era. A follow-up examination by Dr. Bryant one week later seemed to indicate residual tumor in Cleveland's mouth, and a second surgery was recommended. The same cast of characters reassembled on board the *Oneida* for a second, less extensive surgery. Remarkably, Cleveland's condition again remained hidden from the American public. Cancer, an unspoken word in the press until the 1940s because of the universally ominous prognosis it portrayed, was never mentioned during Cleveland's lifetime in relation to his health. During Cleveland's Massachusetts stay, a dentist fashioned a rubber prosthesis to fit and seal the palatal (roof of the mouth) deformity left by the surgery. This allowed Cleveland to speak normally. Later that summer President Cleveland successfully led the political battle to return the United States to a gold standard for American currency. Interestingly, after risking their professional reputations, the operating surgeons believed their efforts would be in vain. Dr. Blair's surgical impression was that Cleveland's tumor was either a sarcoma or squamous carcinoma,[26] both highly lethal malignancies, and would inevitably recur and prove fatal. Cleveland lived 14 more years without cancer recurrence. Details of the surgery did not become public until after his death. Tissue preserved by the College of Physicians of Philadelphia was examined in 1975, and the tumor was determined to be a verrucous carcinoma, a slow-growing, locally spreading cancer, but not a highly invasive or metastasizing cancer. Treatment today would be surgical excision with wide margins, much like what Cleveland received, but hopefully under more favorable operative conditions.

Although Cleveland survived his surgery, most historians believe he failed in his ethical responsibilities. At a time of public crisis, an American president hid his illness and surgery from the American people. He chose personal privacy and political expediency in presidential medi-

---

[26] Squamous cell carcinomas are cancers that arise from the outer layer of the skin. This is the most common cancer of the oral cavity and can often metastasize to local or distant locations early in the disease process. Sarcoma is cancer originating from cells found in the soft tissue parts of the body such as muscles, connective tissues (tendons), blood and lymph vessels, joints and fat. Often local and distant spread occurs early in the disease.

cal issues over any duty to the public trust. In so doing, President Cleveland set a precedent which, unfortunately, has been oft repeated by subsequent presidents.

Woodrow Wilson

The presidency of Woodrow Wilson, the 28th president of the United States, may be the most intriguing in history because it functionally resulted in the first woman president of the United States. Biographers differ regarding Wilson's health as a child. Some describe him as sickly and frail, underdeveloped and unable to participate in sports and physical activity. Others report he was physically fit and participated in horseback riding and baseball. He suspended his schooling twice because of nervous exhaustion, dropping out of Davidson in 1873 and from law school at the University of Virginia in 1880. He was tormented with severe headaches and indigestion throughout his life, the latter which he treated with a stomach pump. But the health problems that impacted his presidency were cardiovascular in etiology.

Wilson was elected president in 1912. Wilson, a Democrat, defeated two former presidents in that election, the incumbent President William H. Taft, who ran as the nominee of the Republican National Party, and former President Teddy Roosevelt, who ran as the nominee of the Bull Moose Party.

Wilson appointed Dr. Cary Grayson, a young naval officer, as his personal physician. The circumstances of Grayson's appointment seem serendipitous. Dr. Grayson in his memoir indicates he was a guest at a luncheon attended by President Wilson in March 1913. During the event Mrs. Ann Howe, Wilson's sister, fell on a staircase and lacerated her forehead. Grayson, who had his equipment at hand, cleaned, sutured and dressed Mrs. Howe's wound. Wilson was so impressed with Grayson's care that three weeks later he appointed him as his personal physician. Although well-educated and personable, the young Grayson had no special professional qualifications or academic appointments for the job, only this chance encounter where the president observed his skills first-hand. Grayson earned Wilson's unqualified trust and became a friend, confidant and advisor to the president. He ultimately impacted Wilson's life and possibly the nation's history as indicated in the following narrative.

In August of 1914, only six days after World War I erupted in Europe, President Wilson's first wife, Ellen, died in the White House of renal failure. At the time of her death the distraught Wilson cried, "Oh, my God, what am I to do?" In truth, Wilson functioned poorly without a mate, and the executive branch of the federal government lacked leadership and efficiency for the next nine months. Dr. Grayson recommended exercise and golf in attempts to cure Wilson's depression, but another action proved more therapeutic. Grayson introduced Edith Galt, a stylish Washington, D.C. widow from Virginia, to President Wilson's cousin, Helen Woodrow Bones, who was serving as the White House hostess. Subsequently, Mrs. Bones introduced Mrs. Galt to President Wilson, and a whirlwind romance evolved. Wilson's energy was restored. He not only became an effective leader of the country and his party, but also carried on an impressive daily romantic correspondence with Mrs. Galt. Wilson and Galt were soon engaged, and then married 16 months after the death of the first Mrs. Wilson. These were scandalous time intervals to many of Washington, D.C. society, especially the Republican congressional opposition.

Edith became the main confidant and advisor of her husband. She was privy to his personal correspondence, as well as classified information. She functioned much like the chief of staff of current administrations. She became an inseparable part of the Wilson presidency even before Wilson's illness.

Early during World War I the United States maintained neutrality. But as Germany sank the "Lusitania" and other ships with American citizens aboard, the United States entrance into World War I became inevitable. In 1916 the Wilsons toured America, promoting war preparedness. Later that year Wilson narrowly won re-election to a second term. In April of 1917 the United States declared war on Germany. On November 11, 1918, a day celebrated yearly as Armistice Day, the defeated German forces agreed to a cessation of hostilities, ending the conflict of World War I.

Wilson is credited with the concept of a League of Nations, the forerunner of the United Nations and a forum for a diplomatic approach to future international disputes. In an address to Congress Wilson stated, "A general association of nations should be formed on the basis of covenants designed to create mutual guarantees of the political independence and territorial integrity of States, large and small equally."

Wilson, who trusted few and delegated poorly, decided that he should be America's emissary to the Paris Peace Conference where surrender terms with Germany and a League of Nations charter were to be debated. With Wilson's leadership the peace treaty and the League of Nations legislation were authored and endorsed by the congress of assembled nations.

Traveling through Europe after the Paris Peace Conference and before returning to America, the Wilsons were treated like royalty. President Wilson was hailed as a conquering hero for his peacemaking efforts. Edith was charming and resplendent in the latest Paris fashions. All that remained was for Wilson to return to the United States and obtain ratification of the Peace Treaty and League of Nations charter by the United States Senate, and his legacy as a peacemaker would be fulfilled. But just as success was at hand, his health failed.

Actually, in addition to his above health problems, Wilson had a long history of episodes suggesting vascular disease. In 1896 at the age of 40 he lost the use of his right hand for several months, possibly a stroke and his first vascular episode. In 1906 at age 50 Wilson developed sudden blindness in the left eye from a retinal hemorrhage and suffered impaired vision for the rest of his life. Hypertension and atherosclerosis were diagnosed by his attending physicians at that time. A second neurologic episode occurred in 1908, causing recurrent paralysis of the right hand. Finally, during the Paris Peace Convention in April 1919, another neurovascular event occurred, causing behavior and cognitive symptoms. His memory failed, his concentration waned and he suffered paranoia. He suspected those around him of spying, especially the French servants. His trusted inner circle, never large at the outset, contracted to his wife Edith, Dr. Grayson, and his secretary of many years, Joseph Tumulty. These episodes suggest Wilson experienced multiple mini-strokes.

Returning to America, Wilson learned that the Senate, with a Republican majority led by Henry Cabot Lodge, did not intend to ratify the peace treaty or the concept of a League of Nations without scrutiny and compromise.[27] The impaired Wilson would not or could not concede

---

[27] The League of Nations charter empowered this organization to keep the international peace and prevent war and aggression. Some of the Republican majority in

any issues. He had forgotten the wisdom of his youth when he had once said, "Uncompromising thought is the luxury of the closeted recluse."

Wilson decided to take his case directly to the American people. He embarked on a whirlwind rail tour across America. Edith, Dr. Grayson and Tumulty were all opposed to the 26-day, 40-speech publicity campaign. All could see that Wilson was a frail and sick man. All tried to persuade him not to undertake the journey. Wilson, however, insisted and none of his inner circle could change his mind. Edith later wrote, "Neither Dr. Grayson nor I could find an answer."

Wilson made it about halfway through the trip. His symptoms were those of heart failure; persistent cough, shortness of breath with activity, followed by frank shortness of breath at rest and when lying down at night. Finally discerning his predicament, Wilson surrendered to his entourage, who were urging him to cancel the campaign. He stated, "I don't seem to realize it, but I seem to have gone to pieces."

On September 26, 1919, one mile outside Wichita, Kansas, Tumulty announced, "The tour is off," due to a "severe nervous attack." Thus began the deception of the country regarding Wilson's health. The tracks were cleared for a 1700-mile dash back to Washington, D.C. Wilson was placed at complete bed rest first on the train, and then back at the White House, and attended by Edith and Dr. Grayson continuously.

But within a week, on October 2, 1919, disaster struck. Wilson slumped in his bathroom, falling off the stool, paralyzed on his entire left side. An air of secrecy immediately enveloped the White House. Access to the president's sick room was limited to Edith, the physicians and servants. Dr. Grayson issued medical bulletins claiming "nervous exhaustion" and "fatigue neurosis," suggesting a functional or psychiatric rather than organic cause of illness, apparently deeming the public

the Senate objected to the League of Nations charter as undermining United States sovereignty, either committing the county to conflicts as peacekeepers or possibly preventing the United States from aggression against other countries to protect its own best interest. Similar issues surfaced recently over United Nations sanctions, United States autonomy and the invasion of Iraq. With Wilson's illness, James M. Cox became the nominee of the Democratic Party in 1920 and ran on a platform that supported the League of Nations charter. He was defeated in a landslide by Warren G. Harding.

disclosure and acceptance greater for the former rather than the latter. His updates were deliberately obtuse, simultaneously suggesting fear but offering hope, counseling no immediate danger but not excluding future danger, offering a good prognosis for complete recovery, but a chance that enforced rest for months would be required. The consultants deferred, publicly at least, to Dr. Grayson's diagnosis and concurred that complete rest was necessary. The media dutifully reported the updates without investigation.

From his perspective, the White House usher, Ike Hoover, later wrote, "Never was deception so universally practiced in the White House as it was in those statements ..." The true nature of Wilson's illness was not disclosed during his presidency.

Grayson and the neurosurgical consultant, Dr. Dercum, also kept private notes. These entries were released by descendants of Dr. Grayson to the public in 1990 and have allowed medical biographers to discern Wilson's true illness. He had a cerebral thrombus (arterial occlusion) affecting the circulation to the right cerebral hemisphere of the brain. He was completely paralyzed on the left side. This involved the left arm, the left leg and the left side of his face.[28] His vision was affected, likely a left homonymous hemianopsia, loss of the left half of his peripheral vision. He was somnolent and, according to his physicians, "seriously disabled, both in a medical and constitutional sense," and, "neither Wilson's thought processes nor his conduct in office would ever be the same again." As to prognosis, "Wilson suffered a devastating trauma, one so extensive that it would be impossible for him to achieve more than a minimal state of recovery."

Apparently the dire circumstances and prognosis were communicated to Mrs. Wilson. Edith insisted that the secrecy be maintained. When Vice President Thomas R. Marshall came to visit, he was turned away. He did not pursue any claim to the presidency for fear of appearing to usurp the office. When the president's cabinet convened a special meet-

---

[28] The neurons (nerve tracts) which originate in the brain cross in the midbrain to the opposite side of the spine and ultimately control the sensory and motor function on the opposite side of the body. Therefore, Wilson's stroke of the right side of the brain caused paralysis on the left side of his face and body.

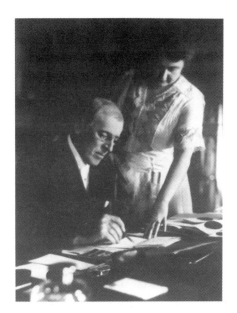

Edith and Woodrow Wilson, the 28th president of the United States, are shown in a posed photograph in 1920 after Wilson's cerebrovascular accident. Notice Wilson's entire left side, which was affected by the stroke, is not seen due to the positioning of President Wilson. Courtesy of Library of Congress Prints and Photographs.

ing four days into the president's illness, Dr. Grayson attended and informed the cabinet that Wilson's mind was not only clear and active, but that the president demanded to know on whose authority the cabinet meeting was assembled and for what purpose. Unable to answer this question, the cabinet adjourned and acquiesced to Dr. Grayson's instructions that only the most urgent matters be brought to the president's attention so that his rest be complete as possible. And so it became implicitly understood that no one would be permitted to take President Wilson's place during his illness.

In Edith Wilson's memoirs, things are presented differently. Rather than relinquish power to the vice president, she remembers being encouraged by the physicians to help her husband through his period of disability by screening all matters and presenting only those of critical importance to him.

With this encouragement, she later wrote of this period, "So began my stewardship. I studied every paper, sent from the different secretaries or senators, and tried to digest and present in tabloid form the things that, despite my vigilance, had to go to the president. I myself never made a single decision regarding the disposition of public affairs. The only decision that was mine was what was important and what was not, and the very important decision of when to present matters to my husband."

So Edith Wilson became the sole liaison between the bedridden president of the United States and Congress and his own cabinet. She controlled access to the president and access became equivalent to power. Functionally, she became the first woman president of the United States. Official documents would be returned with notes in Edith's hand stating, "The President says," followed by Edith's written instructions. When the president's signature was required, his hand was steadied by Edith so he could produce a scribble compared to his normal endorsement.

Between September and November of 1919, 28 bills passed by Congress became law by default because of Wilson's failure to either ratify or veto within the requisite 10 days. Most importantly, Wilson could not advance or debate the League of Nations legislation. This ultimately was rejected by the Senate, and the League of Nations without the United States' participation was never a successful peace-keeping organization.

Wilson was bedridden for six weeks with a varying level of consciousness during that time. He then could be lifted into a wheelchair for short periods of time. Two months after his stroke, a delegation consisting of one Republican and one Democratic senator came to visit, to discern Wilson's condition and fitness for office. (Wilson referred to them as "the Smelling Committee.") Wilson was placed in bed and completely covered except for his face and functioning right arm. The room was poorly lit from the right, and the senators sat on the right. In the 45-minute meeting Wilson's speech and concentration were adequate, and his true physical state was hidden. The "Smelling Committee" was satisfied that the president was competent, and from that point on no further attempts or suggestions of removal from office were entertained.

By four months President Wilson could do limited dictation and would sit in his wheelchair on the White House portico. It was 16 months before he ventured outside the White House. Amazingly, Wilson considered standing for re-election to a third term, to further promote the cause of the League of Nations. He found, appropriately so, little support from his own party.

Wilson survived the remainder of his presidency. He lived an additional two years out of the public eye as a physically and mentally disabled man. It was not until decades later that the American public became aware of the seriousness of his illness and his disability while in office.

Woodrow Wilson had symptoms of atherosclerosis and hypertension many years before his massive cerebrovascular accident. Twenty-first century preventive medications to lower blood pressure and cholesterol levels likely would halve the risk of a stroke. Wilson's stroke ended his advocacy (or ability to compromise) for United States inclusion in the League of Nations. If Wilson's stroke could have been prevented or avoided, chances are high that Wilson and the Senate would have compromised, and the United States would have joined the League of Nations. It is intriguing to consider whether a vigilant League of Nations with the United States of America as a charter and active member could have changed world history. As Arthur Link, a Wilson biographer, put it, "In a world with the United States playing a responsible active role, the possibilities of preventing the rise of Hitler were limitless." Maybe then World War I, the "Great War," the "war to end all wars" would have been just that, rather than a prelude to World War II less than 25 years later.

John F. Kennedy

The deceptions regarding the health of John F. Kennedy, similar to Franklin D. Roosevelt, began well before his political career. Kennedy was never particularly healthy, nor was he healthy in appearance. He entered the Mayo Clinic in the summer of 1934 after his junior year of prep school at Choate. After multiple X-rays and procedures, including sigmoidoscopy, which in those days was accomplished with a rigid 14-inch long scope inserted without sedation through the anus to visualize the colon, his physicians diagnosed diffuse duodenitis and spastic colitis of the bowel. Relapse of his symptoms caused him to withdraw from Princeton in the fall of 1936 and later interrupt his studies at Harvard. His diagnosis remained elusive. Kennedy was treated for jaundice, asthma, colitis and a low blood count. At one time, based on his low blood counts, it was feared that Kennedy might have leukemia.

Kennedy's symptoms paralleled the development of adrenal gland extracts as a treatment for inflammatory conditions. Whether and to what extent Kennedy was prescribed or used adrenal gland extracts prior to 1947 is unknown. Adrenal extracts were usually administered by injection of a liquid suspension or placement of pellets underneath the skin. Kennedy was observed to insert pellets subcutaneously after making an incision in his skin in 1946. Prolonged use of steroids suppresses normal function of the adrenal glands and can lead to atrophy and permanent dysfunction.

In 1940, Kennedy began experiencing back pain, which would trouble him for the remainder of his days. He had intermittent excruciating pain, often precipitated by physical activity that would confine him to bed for days to weeks at a time.

In 1941, with World War II beginning in Europe, despite his medical problems, Kennedy tried to enter military service. He initially failed the physical exams for the Army and Navy officer candidate schools. However, after intervention from his politically connected family, he received a "clean bill of health" and was accepted into Naval Officer training and eventually cleared for sea duty He became commander of a PT boat (patrol-torpedo), a small, maneuverable naval attack boat.

During action in the Solomon Islands, Kennedy's boat, the PT-109, was rammed and sliced in two by a Japanese destroyer. Two shipmates were killed instantly, and Kennedy and the remaining ten crew members were cast into the sea. Although some may question his seamanship, since the PT-109 was the only PT boat rammed during World War II, few can question his heroism after the destruction of his boat. Kennedy rescued several injured shipmates, retrieving them from the sea back to the floating hull of their ship which acted as a life raft. After nine hours in the water, Kennedy organized his crew into swimming parties. The survivors then set out on a five-hour swim to a small atoll. Kennedy swam clutching the straps of an injured comrade's life jacket in his teeth, thus dragging him to safety. He did all this with an unstable back. All 11 men survived.

Kennedy chronicled the adventure of the PT-109 in the book, *Profiles in Courage.* This publication became a bestseller and Pulitzer Prize winner in 1957, and enhanced Kennedy's political prospects.

Shortly after his rescue, recurrence of severe back pain and gastrointestinal symptoms forced Kennedy to seek medical attention. X-rays confirmed a duodenal ulcer. Several consultants recommended back surgery. Kennedy initially opposed surgery, but finally relented. The surgery did not improve Kennedy's pain. The unsuccessful outcome may best be captured by Kennedy's own writing, "In regard to the fascinating subject of my operation, I ... will confine myself to saying that I think the doc should have read just one more book before picking up the saw." All these exploits occurred before any diagnosis of Addison's disease or adrenal insufficiency.

Medical biographers agree that Kennedy had adrenal insufficiency.[29] Although he may have received adrenal extracts intermittently prior, this was clearly diagnosed by physicians during an illness in England in 1947. He was treated with a shot of DOCA (deoxycorticosterone),[30] but still remained quite ill and was given a prognosis of less than a year to live. On the trip home aboard the *Queen Mary,* Kennedy received the last rites of the Catholic Church. He began ongoing treatment with injected or implantable adrenal gland extracts and later oral cortisone when it became available in 1950. Kennedy acquired this disease in a fortunate decade. If Kennedy had developed adrenal insufficiency 10 years earlier when no steroid replacements were available, he would not have survived.

Kennedy positioned himself as the younger, heartier candidate in

---

[29] The adrenal glands are part of the endocrine system of the body, organs which produce hormones important for normal physiologic functions. The body has two adrenal glands, one near the top of each kidney. The glands secrete hormones, such as adrenaline, corticosteroids (cortisol), mineralocorticoids (aldosterone), and some sex hormones (testosterone). These hormones act to regulate blood pressure, fluid balance and electrolyte (sodium and potassium) balance of the body. Adrenal insufficiency (Addison's disease) can cause symptoms of fatigue, muscle weakness, weight loss, nausea, vomiting, diarrhea, salt craving and susceptibility to infection. If untreated, Addison's disease is fatal.

[30] By the 1930s adrenal cortical extract (ACE), obtained from the adrenal glands of healthy domestic animals, was available but not widely recognized as a treatment for Addison's disease. By the early 1940's multiple preparations of ACE and deoxycorticosterone (DOCA), another steroid preparation, were available, all with variable and unregulated potency. Administration was by injection of a suspension or subcutaneous placement of pellets which would, theoretically, gradually dissolve and be absorbed by the body. The Food and Drug Administration removed ACE from the marketplace in the early 1980's because of its inferiority to orally administered synthetic steroid preparations.

the Democratic Party primary in 1960 and claimed the presidency demanded "the strength and health and vigor of ... young men." When the question of Addison's disease was raised by his main opponent for the Democratic Party nomination, Lyndon B. Johnson, Bobby Kennedy, campaign manager for his older brother, responded with a statement that more than shaded the truth: "John F. Kennedy has not, nor has he ever had an ailment described **classically as Addison's disease, which is a tuberculosis destruction of the adrenal gland** ... In the post-war period he had some mild adrenal insufficiency and ... this condition may have arisen out of his wartime experiences of shock and malaria " (bold text added for emphasis by author).

When adrenal insufficiency was initially described by Dr. Addison in the medical literature, the cause described was widespread infection with tuberculosis or fungal pathogens which infiltrated and destroyed the adrenal glands. However, by 1960 the term Addison's disease was synonymous with adrenal insufficiency of all causes with the most common etiology idiopathic in nature. The above statement not only skirted the issue of Addison's disease, but connected Kennedy's infirmities to his World War II heroism. "Mild adrenal insufficiency" is inaccurate since 90 percent loss of adrenal function occurs before clinical symptoms become evident.[31] In retrospect, an article published in the *Archives of Surgery* in 1955, detailing the treatment of Addison's disease (adrenal insufficiency) in patients undergoing back surgery, describes the second back surgery of John F. Kennedy. The hospital, dates of the surgery, patient age, gender and description of the surgery of one of the case histories presented in that article match the public record and news-

---

[31] At the time of Kennedy's autopsy the pathologists directed attention to his adrenal glands. Their findings were published in the *Journal of the American Medical Association* in 1992. No adrenal tissue could be identified on routine gross pathologic examination. Microscopic evaluation of tissue taken from above the kidneys, the normal location of the adrenal glands, revealed only a few individual adrenal cells immersed in a "sea of fat." Findings confirm Kennedy suffered from Addison's disease, likely due to autoimmune destruction of the adrenal glands. However, adrenal atrophy and dysfunction due to excess use of adrenal extracts throughout the late 1930s and 1940s cannot be excluded as the cause of Kennedy's case of Addison's disease.

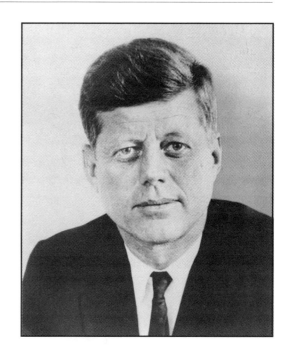

John F. Kennedy, the 35th president of the United States, was the youngest president to occupy the office when he was inaugurated in 1961. Courtesy of Library of Congress Prints and Photographs.

paper accounts of then Senator John F. Kennedy's hospitalization for back surgery.

Kennedy prevailed in the primary against Johnson, selected Johnson as his running mate, and prevailed in the general election to become the youngest elected United States president at 43 years of age. It is paradoxical that Kennedy, an unhealthy candidate, was elected largely because he was viewed as the more hale and vigorous candidate when compared to Richard M. Nixon in the televised debates of the 1960 presidential campaign.

CHAPTER 4

The Assassinations

It is a sad reality that the leading cause of death of American presidents in office is assassination. Four presidents, nine percent of American presidents, have died from wounds inflicted by an assailant's hand. A total of eight presidents have died in office, meaning 50 percent of deaths of presidents in office have been caused by assassination. Since the first attempted assassination of President Andrew Jackson in 1835, there have been at least 12 attacks against eight different presidents. Statistics prove that assassination is an occupational hazard of the American presidency. In this chapter we will concentrate on presidents fatally wounded, the nature of their injuries and the quality and/or effectiveness of medical treatment received.

Abraham Lincoln

Abraham Lincoln, the 16th president of the United States, "Honest Abe," the "Great Emancipator," and by consensus the greatest president in American history, was the first to die by assassination. This is a familiar story, but let's briefly review the historical milestones leading up to Lincoln's assassination and then the details of the injuries and the aftermath of the assassination. Lincoln was elected president in November 1860. He defeated three other opponents, but received only 40 percent of the popular vote. The Republican platform reaffirmed the equality tenets of the Declaration of Independence, advocated the exclusion of slavery from all territories, but upheld states' rights and pledged non-interference in current slave-holding states. Still, only one month after his election in December 1860, South Carolina seceded from the Union. Other states followed, and in February 1861 seven southern states met to form the Confederate States of America. The "house" was divided before Lincoln was inaugurated in March of 1861.

In his inaugural address, Lincoln affirmed his belief that the Union was inviolable by stating, "I therefore consider that ... the Union is unbroken and ... I shall take care, as the constitution itself expressly enjoins upon me, that the laws of the Union be faithfully executed in all the States." Lincoln appealed to the southern states for restraint and reconciliation. He stated, "In your hands, my dissatisfied fellow countrymen, and not in mine, is the momentous issue of civil war. The government will not assail you. You can have no conflict, without being yourselves the aggressors."

The first shots of the Civil War were fired in April of 1861 as Fort Sumter, a Union stronghold in Charleston Harbor, fell to Confederate forces.

For the first two years of the Civil War, little went well for the Union forces. The Battle of Gettysburg in July of 1863 inflicted heavy casualties to both armies, but began to swing the momentum to the North. Lincoln's re-nomination by the Republican Party was not assured until early 1864 when the memories of early embarrassing defeats had been erased by subsequent Union victories and an expectation of an inevitable Union victory. Lincoln was re-elected and began his second term of office in March of 1865. On April 10, 1865, General Lee surrendered at Appomattox and the hostilities of the Civil War ended. Only four days later on April 14, 1865, Lincoln attended an evening performance at Ford's Theatre in Washington, D.C.

So at the time of his theater outing there had been little time for celebration of the end of the Civil War, let alone creation of a firm plan of reconstruction of the South. The Lincolns were accompanied to Ford's Theatre on that fateful evening by Major Henry Rathbone and his fiancée, Clara Harris.[32]

---

[32] General Grant, who accepted General Lee's surrender at Appomattox, was to accompany the president to the theater but reneged under pressure from Mrs. Grant, who did not like the First Lady, Mary Todd Lincoln. Lincoln had settled on Major Rathbone and Ms. Harris as his guests after his invitation to the theater had been declined by fourteen different people. The mercurial and often undignified Mary Lincoln was avoided as a social companion. Rathbone, slashed by Booth's knife during the assassination, was unable to shield the president or prevent Booth's es-

During the play John Wilkes Booth, an actor and a disgruntled southern sympathizer, gained access to Lincoln's box armed with a pistol and a dagger. He fired the pistol from Lincoln's rear at point-blank range, propelling a ball almost one-half inch in diameter with the force of a sledgehammer into the president's brain. Rathbone attempted to restrain Booth, but was slashed in the upper arm by the assassin's knife. Booth leapt from the box to the stage, landed awkwardly, fracturing his left leg, yelled "Sic semper tyrannis" ("thus it shall ever be for tyrants") and hobbled through the wings to make his escape.

A 23-year-old Army surgeon, Dr. Leale, was the first physician to arrive in the presidential box. Lincoln was unconscious with unresponsive pupils. After briefly assuming a knife wound similar to Major Rathbone's injury, Leale located a clot of matted hair on the back of Lincoln's head and the bullet hole in the left occipital bone. On probing this with his fifth finger to a depth of two inches, an oozing of blood flowed from the head wound, and this appeared to improve the irregular and labored breathing of the comatose president. Dr. Leale stated his prognosis, "It is a mortal wound. There is no hope for recovery."

The president was hand-carried to the Peterson house across the street, where Lincoln was placed diagonally because of his height on the bed of an upstairs room, and the death watch began. Ten doctors and 16 men of medicine attended the president during the night, each checking vital signs, many examining and probing the wound with unsterile and ungloved fingers. All reached the same hopeless diagnosis as young Dr. Leale. A probe was used on at least two occasions for further examination and investigation of the wound, once to a distance of over seven inches. Each probing led to an expression of coagulum (semi-clotted blood) from the wound and a brief improvement in the president's respiratory pattern.

The death watch continued throughout the night into the next morning. At 7:22 a.m. on April 15, 1865, respirations stopped and the first

cape. Rathbone despaired over this failure. Eventually, the couple married and moved to Germany. The tragedy of the evening expanded when Rathbone, still anguishing over his failure, in an act suggesting psychosis, killed his wife Clara. He spent the rest of his life in a German asylum for the criminally insane.

president's passing by an assassin's hand was marked by the words of Secretary of War Edwin Stanton, "Now, he belongs to the ages."

An autopsy confined to the head was conducted later that day at the White House. The derringer ball entered the back of the head. It then traversed seven and a half inches through the brain, with the bullet ending in the brain tissue above the eyes in the area of the forehead. There were small bone fragments along the track of the ball. Clotted blood filled the track, and there was mashing of brain tissue surrounding the track and also bleeding into the contiguous brain tissue. This bleeding forced a shift of the brain tissue toward the right side of the skull.

The concussive effects of the bullet, caused by movement of the brain within the rigid skull, resulted in bleeding around the outside of the brain on both sides. There were also fractures of the bony orbits of the eyes from the transmitted concussive force of the ball. (In medical terms, the bullet entered the occipital bone, one inch left of the midline and just above the lateral sinus, which it tore. It traversed the posterior cerebrum, penetrated the left lateral ventricle of the brain, then continued into the anterior cerebrum, where it lodged a distance of seven and a half inches from the entrance wound. The ventricular sinuses of the brain were filled with blood, and there were bilateral subdural hematomas with the right larger than the left. There was a rightward midline shift of the brain. And finally both orbital plates of the frontal bone were fractured with bleeding into both orbits.)

As devastating as this wound was, by 21st century criteria there are a couple of positive prognostic findings of Lincoln's wound:

- Penetrating head injuries with an entry wound only carry a better prognosis than perforating injuries, those both with entry and exit wounds.
- Damage of gunshot wounds to the head are proportionate to kinetic energy (ke) of the missile which is the product of the mass (m) of the bullet and the square of the missile velocity (v), $ke=mv2$. Therefore. the destructive force of a gunshot is most influenced by the bullet's velocity. Handguns are relatively low-energy weapons because they are low velocity weapons.

So the question arises, would Lincoln have had a chance of survival if his assassination occurred today? Remember, James Brady survived a head wound from a handgun during the attempted assassination of Ronald Reagan.

Still, even assuming evaluation and treatment by 21st century neurosurgical techniques, Lincoln would have no chance for meaningful, functional, neurological survival. Modern neurosurgical trauma studies have identified computed tomography (CT) brain scan criteria indicating a poor prognosis for recovery from a head wound. These include:

- Injury to both sides of the brain
- Bleeding inside the skull around the brain
- Shift of the brain to either the left or right or downward within the skull
- Bleeding within the brain of greater than 15 cc (1/2 ounce)

At postmortem examination, Lincoln had all of these findings and thus a very poor prognosis, even by present-day standards.

Finally, by applying the Glasgow Coma Scale, which measures the depth and severity of coma, Lincoln had no chance for meaningful survival. Lincoln, who was immediately and totally unresponsive, would have the lowest score possible, 3 points on the 3 to 15 point scale. In a 1994 study of patients with head wounds, only two patients of a series of 190 patients with Glasgow Coma Scale scores of 3 to 5 points had even a moderately disabled outcome.

Ironically, Lincoln's assassination at the height of his post-war popularity may have preserved his position as the greatest American president in history. Within the last 20 years, in an era of instant media polling, we have seen two presidents achieve maximum popularity post-conflict, but with rapid reversal in the ensuing months. George Bush, Sr. achieved presidential approval ratings of nearly 90 percent in early 1990 following Desert Storm, a campaign to restore freedom to Kuwait after its invasion by neighboring Iraq. But approximately 20 months later he lost his campaign for re-election to Bill Clinton. George W. Bush also transiently enjoyed a spike in presidential approval following the terrorist attack on the World Trade Center buildings and subsequent Afghanistan and Iraq invasions. But at the time of this writing, President Bush has the lowest approval rating recorded for a sitting president since such polling became commonplace.

In post-Civil War times, Lincoln likely would have faced character

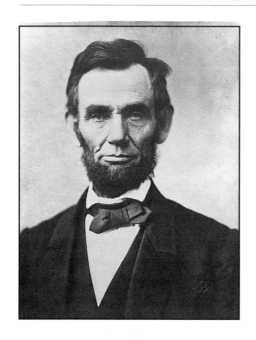

Abraham Lincoln, "Honest Abe," "The Great Emancipator," the 16th president of the United States, is widely acknowledged by historians as America's greatest president. Courtesy of Library of Congress Prints and Photographs.

assassination while trying to reconcile the views of the radical wing of the Republican Party for Reconstruction, views which included confiscation of southern land to pay off war debts, disenfranchisement (no citizenship) for leading Confederate officials, and allowing blacks to vote, with the views of moderate Republicans and favored by the returning Confederate States, which were free election of ex-Confederate officials to government offices, no compensatory damages for Civil War costs and severe restriction of black freedoms and voting rights.

Most historians suggest President Andrew Johnson, who followed Lincoln in office, pursued a lenient plan of reconstruction similar to that favored by Lincoln. Remember what happened to President Johnson. He conflicted with the radical wing of the Republican Party, became the first president to be impeached, and barely avoided conviction and expulsion from the presidency by a single vote in the Senate.

Surely Lincoln would not have survived the post-Civil War presidency without scars, but in my estimation he deserves the recognition as America's greatest president. This self-educated and self-made man derived his opinions from intense study, thought and debate rather than a pre-determined belief system. Even after forming an opinion, he remained empathetic to his opponents, a trait which served his political career well. Lincoln proclaimed slavery "an injustice and bad policy" and contradictory to the Declaration of Independence which states, "all men are created equal." He did not invoke the more divisive divine or "higher power" argument to the slavery question as did many abolition-ists of his time. Lincoln did not believe the Constitution gave the gov-ernment the right to abolish slavery in states where the practice was established and supported by the laws of that state. In a time of discor-dant views severe enough to initiate warfare, Lincoln perceived that America's strength was its diversity and that its strength could only be achieved by preservation of the Union, rather than separation into geo-graphical provinces. Lincoln abhorred war and maintained only preser-vation of the Union and the promise of America could justify the con-flict. His heartfelt challenge contained in his famous Gettysburg Ad-dress, personally written for the dedication of a cemetery for Civil War casualties, captures the essence of the man. It reads in part:

"The world will little note, nor long remember, what we say here, but it can never forget what they did here. It is for us, the living, rather, to be dedicated here to the unfinished work which they who fought here, have, thus far, so nobly advanced. It is rather for us to be here dedicated to the great task remaining before us — that from these honored dead we take increased devotion to that cause for which they here gave the last full measure of devotion — that we here highly resolve that these dead shall not have died in vain — that this nation, under God, shall have a new birth of freedom — and that, government of the people, by the people, for the people, shall not perish from the earth."

As opposed to most presidential deaths where conspiracies were fabricated, Lincoln's death involved a conspiracy with John Wilkes Booth as the chief conspirator and ultimate assassin. After initial plans to kid-nap and hold Lincoln as ransom for lenient southern treatment failed, the conspirators deemed assassination a more attainable goal.

At virtually the same time Lincoln was assassinated, an accomplice, Lewis Powell, attacked the bedridden Secretary of State William Seward who had been injured a week earlier in a carriage accident. Powell slashed Seward and several household members with a knife. Although seri-ously injured, Seward survived.

A second accomplice, George Atzerodt, was assigned the task of assassinating Vice President Andrew Johnson. Atzerodt fortified himself for the task at a local tavern, but became intoxicated and thus failed to carry out his assignment.

Among the other accomplices were David Herold, who accompanied Booth on his escape through Maryland and Virginia, and Mary Surratt, who owned the boarding house where the plot was hatched, but likely had no personal knowledge of the conspiracy.

Booth fractured his leg leaping from Lincoln's box to the stage at Ford's Theatre, but still escaped Washington, D.C. into the Maryland countryside. There his leg was set by Dr. Samuel Mudd. Booth then fled in a serpentine course across the Potomac into Virginia where, 12 days after the assassination, he was discovered, trapped in a barn and finally shot and killed.

Ultimately, Powell, Atzerodt, Herold and Mary Surrratt were hanged. Others, including Dr. Samuel Mudd, were sentenced to life in prison at hard labor. Dr. Mudd, a Maryland farmer, had not practiced medicine in years when Booth appeared on his doorstep the day after the assassination. Although Mudd had met Booth previously, he claimed not to recognize Booth with a beard. It is unlikely that Mudd was aware of Lincoln's assassination when he set Booth's leg. (Remember these were times long before CNN and instant news access.) Mudd was arrested and charged when the boot cut from Booth's leg with Booth's initials engraved was found at Mudd's farm. Mudd maintained his innocence, but was convicted. Mudd became a model prisoner. In August of 1867 when an outbreak of yellow fever claimed the life of the prison's doctor, Mudd offered his services and saved the lives of soldiers and prisoners alike. On the recommendation of prison officials, Mudd was pardoned by President Andrew Johnson and released from prison in 1869.

Mudd's involvement in the Lincoln assassination led to the origination of the colloquialism, "His name is Mudd," a moniker which Mudd's descendants have continued to endure. The family has continued to maintain Dr. Mudd's innocence and also the ethical duty of a physician to treat the sick or injured who seek his/her care. With legislative support, the family received a letter from President Jimmy Carter in 1979, 114 years after the Lincoln assassination, which read in part:

"The circumstances of the surgical aid of the escaping assassin and the imputed concealment of his flight are deserving of the lenient construction, as within the obligations of professional duty and thus inadequate evidence of a guilty sympathy with the crime of a criminal. I am hopeful that these conclusions will be given widespread circulation which will restore dignity to your grandfather's name and clear the Mudd family name of any negative connotation or implied lack of honor."

James A. Garfield

Only 15 years later, a second American president was the victim of assassination. James Garfield was the compromise candidate of the Republican Party in 1880, nominated on the 36th ballot of the Republican Party convention. Surprisingly, he won the election and became the 20th president of the United States in 1881. Garfield had been president only a few months when he was shot in the back with a .44 caliber revolver from approximately five feet at the Washington, D.C. train station.

From the assassination onward Garfield, as stated by the authors of *Medical Cover-ups in the White House,* was "a victim of his doctors … (His) death included all the worst elements that could be found in a presidential medical crisis: faulty diagnosis, grossly improper treatment, prideful bickering among doctors and a massive cover-up of the truth before and after death."

Shortly after the shooting, Dr. Bliss arrived on the scene and assumed care. Garfield was pale and bradycardic (slow heart rate). Dr. Bliss discovered the entry wound in the back, four inches right of the spine at the level of the 11th rib. He used his finger and a probe, both without any attempts at sterility, but "with great caution" to examine the wound. Subsequent events indicate that he created a false channel with his probings that proceeded forward or anteriorly into the abdomen. He was able to palpate the spongy surface of the liver with his finger. He surmised the bullet had passed along this same route into the abdomen and through the liver and that Garfield would soon die from intra-abdominal hemorrhage.

In actuality, the bullet struck and shattered the right 11th rib in the right lower back, deflected medially and passed obliquely from right to left through the body of the first lumbar vertebra, and entered the abdominal cavity on the **left** side of the spine, where it severed some small mesenteric arteries (vessels supplying the membranes supporting the bowel) and injured the splenic (spleen) artery before coming to rest in the area of the pancreas. None of the bullet's path was appreciated pre-mortem other than the rib fracture.[33]

Garfield surprised the doctors by not only surviving the night, but for 80 unpleasant days. Multiple additional examinations with unclean fingers, instruments and catheters failed to locate the bullet. Alexander Graham Bell, the inventor of the telephone, was recruited to use his electronics as a primitive metal detector, to try to locate the bullet's position. His efforts were unsuccessful. Apparently the metal springs in Garfield's bed prevented Bell's equipment from functioning optimally.

Also Garfield's illness and confinement in the summer heat and humidity of Washington, D.C. initiated construction of the first working air-conditioner. Navy engineers devised a system to pump air cooled by blocks of ice through cotton filters to remove humidity into the bedridden president's room. With some trial and error, this eventually successfully lowered the temperature in Garfield's sick room *(see cover)* to a steady 77 degrees from the ambient 90-degree heat of the Washington, D.C. summer.

Despite European acceptance by the 1880s of the germ theory of infection and aseptic technique for surgery, these medical advances were in their infancy in America, practiced only in parts of New England. Unfortunately for Garfield, the germ theory had not been accepted or integrated into the medical community of Washington, D.C. in 1881.

Garfield underwent two operations to explore and expand the en-

---

[33] The physicians involved in President Garfield's care published an account of the care of the dying president in the *Journal of American Medicine* in 1901. Interestingly, there were clinical clues to the true path of the bullet. Garfield, while still at the train station, "complained very much of a sense of weight and heaviness" in his legs. After transfer to the White House, the physicians chronicled that Garfield "complains of spasmodic pains in the extremities … which he describes as shooting up the legs toward the body." In retrospect, these symptoms were neurologic in character, indicating involvement of the spinal cord due to the course of the bullet medially through the vertebral body. Since these symptoms abated during the course of Garfield's illness, likely the symptoms resulted from temporary spinal cord pressure due to hemorrhage or bony fragments. Still, the true course of the bullet was not appreciated prior to autopsy.

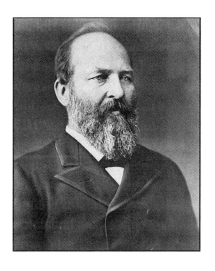

James A. Garfield, the 20th president of the United States, was a dark horse candidate of the Republican Party. He was probably the most unlikely president ever elected to the White House. Courtesy of Library of Congress Prints and Photographs.

trance gunshot wound during the ensuing months, draining new abscess pockets and removing bits of clothing and rib. Finger and flexible catheter explorations of the wound were liberally employed to drain infection. Garfield's fevers worsened. He developed symptoms and signs of generalized infection, septicemia or bacteria in the bloodstream, with secondary abscesses in both axillae (armpits) and right parotid gland (salivary gland often swollen with mumps). He became delirious. His nutrition and hydration were maintained with liquid foods and nutrient enemas. Garfield lost over 75 pounds during his 80-day confinement.

On September 19, 1881, Garfield complained of sudden chest pain and died rapidly. The autopsy the next day showed the bullet path as previously described. The cause of death was fresh intra-abdominal hemorrhage, apparently from rupture of a pseudo-aneurysm[34] of the splenic

---

[34] Aneurysm, a term usually used in referring to blood vessels, indicates an abnormal dilatation of the blood vessel wall. Although the vessel wall is dilated, it is intact. Aneurysms increase susceptibility of arteries to rupture and bleed. A pseudo-aneurysm is an apparent dilatation of a blood vessel, but where the vessel wall is not entirely intact. What prevents bleeding is clot or fibrous tissue surrounding the blood vessel. Pseudo-aneurysms are even more susceptible to bleeding as disruption of the clot often occurs. In Garfield's case, the initial bullet path probably pierced the artery to the spleen, but clotting around the vessel prevented exsanguination. Death occurred 80 days later when the clot dam broke and allowed resumption of internal bleeding. He certainly would have died from infection if recurrent bleeding had not occurred first.

artery injured at the time of the shooting. But there was also a 20-inch-long subcutaneous (underneath the skin) abscess tract stretching from the initial wound entry site at the 11th rib almost to the crest of the right hip bone. Also an orange-sized, right intra-abdominal abscess was found between the liver and the large bowel. These infected areas were clearly related to the physicians' multiple, unsterile examinations. Some have even suggested the splenic aneurysm could have been related to spread of infection rather than Garfield's initial traumatic injuries. Likely, Garfield's infection, although a fatal illness in its own right, did not cause Garfield's final demise. Certainly the infection, resulting from or complicated by his physicians' treatments, contributed to the agony of his illness.

Perhaps the most ironic indictment of the physicians' care came from Garfield's crazed assassin, Charles Guiteau. In a moment of lucidity at his trial, he shouted, "[I] admit the shooting of the president, but not the killing. The doctors did that." He was hanged for his crime, but his assertions are not entirely unfounded. Today with 21st century trauma care, diagnostic tests to locate the exact injuries, modern surgical care and antibiotics to battle infection, Garfield almost certainly would survive.

Garfield was incapable of presidential leadership during his prolonged illness. Vice President Chester Arthur stayed out of Washington, D.C.[35] so as not to appear too eager to assume power. The United States

---

[35] The Republican Party National Convention of 1880 had three viable candidates for the presidential nomination: Former President Ulysses S. Grant, the favorite of the Stalwart branch of the Party, Senator James G. Blaine from Maine, and John Sherman, "favorite son" candidate from Ohio and the candidate supported by Garfield. The largest plurality of the factions belonged to the Stalwart (Grant) wing, but the Stalwarts could never muster a majority required for nomination. When Garfield was nominated, it became imperative for Republican Party unity that a member of the Stalwart faction be named as the vice presidential nominee. Chester A. Arthur was that candidate. Charles Guiteau, the assassin, was a member of the Stalwart wing of the Republican Party. He supported the Garfield/Arthur ticket. He wrote a speech in support of the candidates, but never delivered it. In Guiteau's deluded mind, that undelivered address was largely responsible for Garfield's election. Therefore, Guiteau believed he deserved a position of prestige and patronage in the new administration and became disgruntled when an appointment was not forthcoming. After the

was leaderless for an extended period for the first, but not the last time, because of an incapacitated president. No legislation to establish protocol for transfer of power during presidential disability was considered.

William McKinley

Only 20 years later, a third American president, William McKinley, the 25th president of the United States, was murdered by an assassin. William McKinley, like William H. Harrison, James Garfield and Warren Harding, was a native of Ohio who became president and who died in office.

McKinley was elected to Congress in 1876. Early in his political career he was an isolationist and protectionist, convinced that cheap imported goods would threaten American jobs and salaries. Passage of the McKinley Tariff Act of 1890, taxing imported agricultural and manufactured goods, propelled McKinley to national notoriety.

During his presidency, somewhat ironically, McKinley presided over a period of unprecedented American global expansion. Cuba, Puerto Rico and the Philippine Islands all became American protectorates as a result of the Spanish-American War and Hawaii was annexed by Congress. It was also a time of unparalleled industrial expansion.

In his last speech at the Pan-American Exposition in 1901 in Buffalo, New York, McKinley, the isolationist and protectionist, acknowledged that America's industrial growth forced a new openness to global commerce, "Our capacity to produce has developed so enormously, and our products have so multiplied, that the problem of more markets requires our urgent and immediate attention."

The next day McKinley was shot while shaking hands in a reception line at the Exposition on September 6, 1901. Leon Czolgosz fired two bullets at point-blank range from a revolver he had concealed in a bandaged hand. The first bullet struck a button on McKinley's suit and did not penetrate the skin. The second bullet entered the abdomen.

---

assassination, Guiteau was widely quoted from his writings in the press declaring, "I am a Stalwart, and Arthur will be president." Thus Arthur, truly anguished over Garfield's shooting, was tarnished by the political affiliation of the mentally unstable assassin. He wisely remained in New York until Garfield's death.

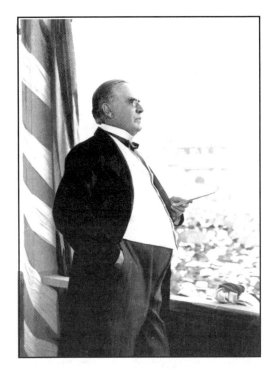

William McKinley, the 25th president of the United States, pictured delivering his last address at the Buffalo Exposition just days before his assassination. Courtesy of the Ohio Historical Society.

McKinley was moved to a small, poorly equipped hospital on Exposition grounds and underwent immediate surgery. Aseptic technique, now standard medical practice, was employed. The president's abdomen was washed, then bathed with a chloride solution and draped with sterile towels. The surgical team prepped similarly and wore steam-sterilized gowns. In contrast to modern surgery, the surgeons operated with bare hands, as surgical gloves were not yet in use. The surgical team, however, faced several problems.

First, McKinley was corpulent and, as the picture shows, had a central distribution of his adiposity. The surgeons had to work through a three-inch layer of abdominal fat to access the abdominal cavity. They had no surgical retractors to aid their task. Second, the surgeons were primarily dependent on natural light to illuminate the surgical field, and at five p.m. in Buffalo, New York, in September, the light was failing. The head surgeon, Dr. Matthew D. Mann, commented that it was like operating at "the darkened end of a big hole."

Surgical findings indicated that the bullet had entered the left upper abdomen five and one-half inches below the left nipple and one and a half inches left of the midline. It then perforated both the anterior and posterior walls (front and rear walls) of the stomach along the greater curvature of that viscera. Both holes in the stomach were repaired by oversewing of the wounds. The bullet's course behind the stomach could not be discerned as further search for the bullet was halted when the manipulation of McKinley's stomach and intestines adversely affected his vital signs.[36] The abdomen was copiously irrigated with a saline solution, but no drains were left in place.

McKinley survived for eight days after his surgery. He received fluids through retention enemas, morphine for pain and digitalis for a fast heart rhythm. Although he had a low grade fever, there were no overt findings of infection. The doctors, both surgeons and additional consultants, thought McKinley's prognosis was favorable and relayed this information to Vice President Teddy Roosevelt who was keeping vigil. Thus assured, Roosevelt departed Buffalo on September 10 for a hiking trip in the Adirondack Mountains. However, McKinley's status worsened, and he died three days later on September 13, 1901. By this time, Vice President Roosevelt was in parts unknown in the Adirondacks, and mountain rangers had to be dispatched on foot to find and inform Roosevelt of the president's death.

At the postmortem examination conducted on McKinley, the stomach sutures placed to close the bullet holes through the walls of the stomach were intact, but there was necrosis (non-viability or death) of the surrounding stomach tissue, which appeared ready to slough (separate from the living tissue, thus reopening the wounds of the stomach wall). There was extensive necrosis along the track of the ball which

---

[36] The details of McKinley's surgery and care were recounted by his physicians in the *Journal of the American Medical Association* in October 19, 1901. A mirror was used to try and direct the natural light unto the surgical field. Toward the end of the operation, an electric light with reflector was put into use. McKinley's hemodynamic status was monitored by the rate, amplitude and character of his pulse. The blood pressure cuff did not become available for over another decade. The use of a cuff and stethoscope to determine blood pressure was first described by Nicolai Korotkoff in Russia in 1905, four years after McKinley's surgery. The characteristic sounds heard with the stethoscope over the artery distal to the cuff as one lowers the pressure in the blood pressure cuff, which identify the systolic and diastolic pressure readings, are still referred to as Korotkoff sounds.

extended behind the stomach and involved portions of the pancreas,[37] left kidney and extended to the retro-peritoneal adipose tissue, the soft tissues of the inner back. Although extensively sought, the location of the bullet was not found. There were no exit wounds.

The pathologists presumed the bullet remained hidden in the ample fatty stores in McKinley's back.

The cause of death was shock due to the extensive tissue necrosis. Likely, the stomach and pancreatic injury led to leakage of gastric and pancreatic secretions into the abdominal cavity, causing inflammation, pancreatitis and resulting tissue necrosis. This likely precipitated massive fluid loss into the abdominal cavity, with resulting hypotension, shock and death. McKinley would likely survive his wounds today with the availability of current diagnostics, trauma and surgical skills, intravenous fluid replacement and potent antibiotics to prevent or cure infections. Any observed pancreatic injury by pre-operative or intra-operative techniques would warrant placement of temporary abdominal drains to prevent fluid accumulation and possible toxicity.

The industrial development and global expansion of the country during McKinley's tenure created the foundation for the emergence of the United States of America as an international power. Under the guidance of the progressive Teddy Roosevelt, and later Woodrow Wilson, America achieved this distinction during the first 20 years of the 20th century.

After McKinley's death, the third assassination of an American president in 36 years, the Secret Service was formed. There has subsequently been only one successful assassination in the last 100 years.

John F. Kennedy

That assassination, of course, was John F. Kennedy. Even though this occurred 40 years ago, most individuals of the Baby Boomer gen-

---

[37] The pancreas is an organ which sits behind the stomach. Its main function is the production of enzymes which it secretes into the small bowel, facilitating digestion. If the pancreas becomes injured or inflamed (pancreatitis), these enzymes are released inside the abdomen, chemically harming the stomach, bowel and support structures of the abdomen.

eration and older remember their exact circumstances when first hearing the news of Kennedy's shooting. This was the first assassination attempt to occur during the era of television, which greatly expanded the reported details of the shooting, death and funeral of Kennedy, and also the specifics of the manhunt, capture, shooting and death of Kennedy's assassin, Lee Harvey Oswald. Multiple, complex and persistent conspiracy theories exist in spite of the conclusions of the Warren Commission, i.e., Kennedy was murdered by a lone gunman.

From a medical standpoint, the findings are straightforward. Kennedy was shot while riding in his motorcade through Dealey Plaza in Dallas, Texas. That lone gunman, as determined by the Warren Commission, was Lee Harvey Oswald, who fired from the sixth floor of the Texas School Book Depository Building. Kennedy was rushed to the emergency room at Parkland Medical Center, but could not be saved. Rather than perform the autopsy in Texas, the president's body was flown back to Washington, D.C. where the postmortem examination was conducted. There is an immense amount of material written about the Kennedy assassination, but we are going to rely on the three pathologists who did the autopsy. After a 29-year reticence to discuss the topic, the three pathologists involved in President Kennedy's autopsy were interviewed and their statements published in the Journal of the American Medical Association in 1992. The pathologists were James Joseph Humes, MD, "J" Thornton Boswell, M.D., and Pierre Finck, M.C., all military physicians. The site of the autopsy, Bethesda Naval Medical Center, may have been chosen by the family because of Kennedy's naval service.

Kennedy was struck by two bullets. Although the sequence of the injuries was not evident from autopsy findings alone, other evidence available, primarily the home video filmed by Abraham Zapruder, indicates the sequence of the wounds. The first entered the upper back to the right of the spine, at the right base of the neck. This bullet exited in the anterior neck right below the tracheal cartilage (Adam's apple) in the midline. In fact, during the emergency room resuscitative efforts a tracheotomy was performed to place a breathing tube and the incision into the trachea actually was made over the location of the exit wound. The tracheotomy incision initially obscured the location of the exit wound from the pathologists on external inspection. Questioning of the surgeons involved in Kennedy's emergency room care confirmed the presence of an exit wound in the anterior neck when Kennedy was initially evaluated in the Emergency Department. The neck wound was not a fatal wound. Ironically, Kennedy's chronic back pain, unrelieved by his two previous back surgeries, may have played a role in his death. Kennedy wore a rigid metal back brace, which may have kept him more erect after the first wound and thus exposed his head to the second fatal injury.

The second wound was a fatal head shot. From the time this bullet struck Kennedy, there was no hope for recovery. The bullet entered the back of the skull through the right occipital bone and exited the right anterior head, exploding away almost two-thirds of the right cerebrum (the front lobe of the brain and the repository of memory, speech and personality). What may give rise to conspiracy theories is the layman belief that the injury should be greatest at the site of entry of a head wound. But actually the more typical pattern related to ballistics is a small wound at entry and an explosive exit wound, which is exactly what Kennedy suffered. As previously mentioned, damage of gunshot wounds to the head are proportionate to kinetic energy of the missile, which is most influenced by the missile velocity (see Chapter 4). Rifles, as opposed to handguns, are high velocity weapons and impart a far greater energy and destructive force to their target. The pathologist's opinion was "two bullets from the rear." A major factor in their opinion was the appearance at the entry and exit wounds. A missile through the mantle of the skull bone creates a larger area of damage on the exit side of the skull bone, similar to the cratering effect seen from a BB piercing a window. This crater effect was seen on the inside mantle of the back part of the skull, indicating an entrance wound and, on the outside mantle of the right front of the skull indicating an exit wound. The anterior skull had to be reconstructed from the multiple scattered fragments of bone retrieved at the crime scene.

The pathologists all concurred in their opinions. The evidence from the postmortem examination "provides irrefutable proof that the president was struck by only two bullets that came from above and behind from a high velocity weapon which caused the fatal wounds." They also expressed confidence that the Warren Commission findings were correct and applied terms such as "hoax," "smear" and "pure fiction" to the many publications advancing conspiracy theories regarding Kennedy's assassination. Dr. Humes, the chief pathologist, stated, "My orders were to find the cause of death, and I was told to get anyone I thought necessary to help do the autopsy, but to limit it to only the help I needed. Hell, I could have called in people from Paris or Rome if I thought it necessary, but as it turned out, I didn't." The nature of Kennedy's wounds and cause of death were self-evident.

Kennedy initially was deified by the American public as a great American president, martyr and hero. Subsequent revelations of marital infidelity and misrepresentation of health concerns have tarnished the Kennedy reputation. To historians, the Bay of Pigs incident in Cuba, continued Cold War tensions and construction of the Berlin Wall, brewing conflict in southeast Asia, and shortcomings in civil rights issues constrain their ratings of the Kennedy presidency. Lyndon B. Johnson, Kennedy's rival for the Democratic Party presidential nomination but the ultimate vice presidential candidate, inherited the presidency during the turbulent decade of the 1960s. Civil rights issues, the Cold War and the Vietnam War also vexed Johnson's years in office. Still, in the most recent poll of presidential leadership, Johnson surprisingly rates a slight edge over Kennedy.

CHAPTER 5

The Attempted Assassinations

FORTUNATELY, MOST ASSASSINATION attempts have been un-successful. One such attempt was thwarted by modern trauma care.

Ronald Reagan

President Ronald Reagan, who at the age of 70 years was the oldest elected American president,[38] was shot 70 days after assuming office in 1981 as he walked to his limousine following a Washington, D.C. speech.[39] Ironically, the bullet which struck the president ricocheted off his limousine, which was armor-plated for his protection.

---

[38] At 93 years of age, Ronald Reagan is also the American president who lived to the oldest age. Ronald Reagan retired from public life in 1994 with his declaration by letter of his diagnosis of Alzheimer's syndrome and these words: "I now begin the journey that will lead me into the sunset of my life. I know that for America there will always be a bright dawn ahead. Thank you, my friends. May God always bless you." He lived in quiet seclusion until his death in 2004.

Previously, John Adams, the second president of the United States, held this distinction. He was born in 1735 and died at 92 years of age in 1826.

Gerald Ford, now 93 years old, may pass Ronald Reagan as the president surviving to the oldest age in November 2006. He suffered a brain stem cerebrovascular accident during the 2000 Republican Party National Convention, but reportedly had a good recovery. Public interviews in June 2004 suggest he remains active with swimming and golf. However, he appears frail and did not attend the 2004 Republican National Convention or the inauguration ceremonies for George W. Bush's second term in January of 2005.

Jimmy Carter, at age 81, remains active in political and humanitarian pursuits. He has no reported health issues.

George H. W. Bush, now 82 years old, celebrated his 80th birthday by going skydiving. Although he has required treatment for hyperthyroidism (an overactive thyroid gland) and atrial fibrillation (an irregular heart rhythm), he remains active and in good health.

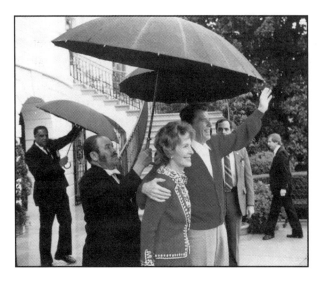

President and Nancy Reagan arriving back at the White House after discharge from the hospital following the president's gunshot wound and surgery. Courtesy of Library of Congress Prints and Photographs.

At the sound of gunfire, the head of the Secret Service detail hurled President Reagan into the limousine. As the limousine sped toward the White House, Reagan coughed hard, and frothy blood appeared in the palm of his hand. The Secret Service agent, in what may have been a life-saving decision, immediately diverted the limousine to George Washington University Medical Center nine blocks away.

On arrival only 10 minutes after the shooting, Reagan walked into the emergency room complaining of shortness of breath, then slumped to his knees. His initial blood pressure was 80 mmHg by palpation. Normal systolic pressure is 120 mmHg, and low blood pressure in the circumstance of acute blood loss may herald shock. He was rapidly ad-

---

[39] Reagan was struck by a bullet fired from a handgun by John Hinckley. Three other people in the president's entourage were hit by bullets, Press Secretary James Brady, Secret Service agent Timothy McCarthy, and Washington, D.C. police officer Thomas Delahanty. Ultimately all survived. James Brady was the most seriously injured with a head wound. He survived with modern neurosurgery, but with significant disability. In 1993, President Reagan signed into law the Brady Handgun Violence Prevention Act (The Brady Bill) which mandated a criminal background check and a five-day waiting period for those purchasing handguns through licensed dealers. It was later struck down by the Supreme Court as an "unfunded mandate" imposed on the states. Today an "instant" check system developed by the Federal Bureau of Investigation is operative. A three-day wait is required if the system cannot immediately approve or deny an applicant.

ministered oxygen, type O Rh-negative (uncrossmatched) blood and intravenous crystalloid fluids. An oblong, one-and-a-half-centimeter-long entrance wound with minimal subcutaneous air (air which has leaked from the lungs into the soft tissues of the chest) was noted in the left posterior axillary line at the fourth intercostal space (underneath the left armpit). Interestingly, at the time of surgery it was determined that the bullet had been flattened into the shape of a dime when it first struck the armor-plated limousine and entered the president on edge, leaving a relatively small and unobtrusive entrance wound.

A chest tube[40] yielded 1200 cc. of bloody drainage and persistent drainage of 200 to 300 cc. every 15 minutes. Normal total body blood volume is 5,000 to 6,000 cc, so Reagan had lost approximately 20 percent of his blood volume on arrival at the hospital.

Rapid loss of 33 percent of blood volume can precipitate fatal shock.[41] A portable chest X-ray showed partial re-expansion of the lung, a hazy infiltrate (fluid collection) in the left lower lobe of the lung and a metallic fragment at the level of the 10th thoracic vertebra superimposed on the left heart border. (An X-ray is a two-dimensional picture. The bullet fragment was behind the heart.)

Because of the continued blood loss through the chest tube, Dr. Benjamin Aaron, Chief of Thoracic Surgery, determined that chest exploration was needed to stem the bleeding. On being informed of this decision, Reagan said to the surgeons, "Please tell me you're all Republicans." Dr. Giordano, one of the surgeons and a liberal Democrat, re-

---

[40] The outer surface of the lung is covered by a membrane called the pleura. This membrane also lines the inside of the chest wall. Between these membranes is the pleural space, which under healthy conditions is only a potential space. However, if fluid or blood accumulates in this space, the resulting pressure of the fluid can compress or collapse the air-filled lung, which compromises breathing. A chest tube can be placed through a small incision in the chest wall into the pleural space to drain fluid or blood and re-expand the lung.

[41] Shock is a state where adequate blood flow to internal organs to maintain normal function fails. In acute blood loss, there is insufficient fluid volume remaining in the vascular space (arteries and veins) to allow the heart to maintain normal blood flow. Much like a well going dry, the pump, although working, cannot do its job of delivering water if there's no water to pump.

plied, "Today, Mr. President, we are all Republicans."

Only 80 minutes after being shot, Reagan received anesthesia. At surgery, reconstruction of the bullet's path indicated that it glanced off the top of the seventh rib, posteriorly (toward the back). It then traversed the left lower lobe of the lung, coursing three and a half inches to the medial or middle edge of the lung surface. The bullet came to rest one inch from the heart and aorta. Injury of either of these structures would have caused massive bleeding. Although the bullet was flattened to the size of a dime, the extensive lung tissue injury suggested that the missile took a tumbling and thus more destructive path through the lung. Reagan was transfused with a total of eight units of blood (4,000 cc. of blood) before and during surgery. Over all, he lost 3,400 cc. of blood, over half his normal blood volume.

Reagan's post-operative course, considering he was a 70-year-old man with a bullet wound to the chest, was relatively benign. He was extubated (breathing tube removed) and transferred from the intensive care unit within 24 hours. He underwent bronchoscopy[42] post-operatively for the removal of lung secretions from the airways to aid breathing and again several days later for persistent hemoptysis (coughing up blood). He received narcotics for pain. He had some post-operative disorientation, enough to concern Mrs. Reagan. He developed a fever of 102 degrees. Antibiotics were administered, although no clear infection was identified. He slowly improved and was discharged just short of two weeks after the shooting. He returned to a limited schedule, initially working one to two hours a day. He worked his first full day eight weeks after the attack and announced that he was fully recovered at a press conference one week after that. His physician later admitted that full recovery took approximately six months.

Reagan was the first president wounded by a gunshot while in office to survive. Clearly, his wound was life-threatening. With hypotension (low blood pressure) 10 minutes after the injury, even a reasonably

---

[42] Bronchoscopy employs a flexible tube with fiber-optics to obtain direct visualization of the major bronchi, breathing tubes, of the lungs. Bronchoscopy can be helpful in diagnosis of chest masses, or hemoptysis (bleeding from the lungs) or in treatment, especially the removal of secretions as employed post-operatively during President Reagan's recovery.

short delay in care could have precipitated irreversible, hypovolemic shock *(see footnote 41)*. If afforded only the medical care available to assassinated Presidents Garfield and McKinley, Reagan's fate would have been similar. The 20th century trauma care administered to Reagan stands in stark contrast to the limited, even harmful care available to previous presidents only 80 to 100 years earlier.

Theodore Roosevelt

Teddy Roosevelt was the victim of an assassination attempt after his tenure in office, but while a candidate again for the office of president of the United States. Roosevelt was a member of the Republican Party when he assumed the presidency on the death of William McKinley in 1901 and when elected to his own term in 1904. In 1912 after four years out of the White House, Roosevelt ran for president as the third party nominee of the Bull Moose Party against incumbent William Howard Taft, the candidate of the Republican Party, and Woodrow Wilson, the Democratic Party candidate.

Roosevelt was scheduled to give an evening speech at the civic auditorium in Milwaukee on October 14. Roosevelt exited his hotel, entered and stood in an open car acknowledging the crowd, when a shot rang out. Roosevelt did not think he had been hit, but on the drive to the auditorium noticed blood on his shirt. The bullet, fortunately, passed through the manuscript of his speech, which was 50 pages in length and folded over in his coat, and also through a metal spectacle case before striking Roosevelt in the right chest. On arrival at the auditorium, he was examined by his personal physician and advised to cancel the speech. Roosevelt refused. As the wound was dressed, a local Bull Moose leader informed the crowd that Roosevelt had been shot.

Roosevelt was assisted onto the platform and began speaking, "I do not care a rap about being shot, not a rap." He then unbuttoned his coat to show his blood-stained shirt. "I'm going to ask you to be very quiet and please excuse me from making a very long speech. I'll do the best I can, but you see there is a bullet in my body … but it takes more than a bullet to kill a Bull Moose." The crowd cheered wildly. Roosevelt, encouraged by the crowd's response, spoke for 50 minutes.

After the speech he was examined at a local hospital. The entrance

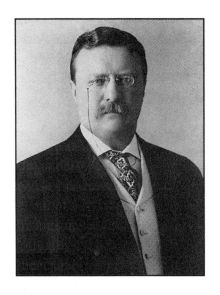

Theodore Roosevelt, the 26h president of the United States, presided during America's industrial revolution and growth into a world power. Roosevelt is memorialized with Presidents Washington, Jefferson and Lincoln on Mount Rushmore in South Dakota. Courtesy of Library of Congress Prints and Photographs.

wound was just to the right and an inch below the right nipple. There was no exit wound. X-rays indicated the bullet burrowed underneath the skin three inches superiorly and medially (upward and toward the middle) through the soft tissues of the chest wall, but had not entered the pleural space (lung cavity). No probing or surgery was done.

Roosevelt was transferred to Chicago and hospitalized for eight days. He then traveled home to New York by train. His campaigning was virtually over. A month later he placed second to Woodrow Wilson in the presidential election of 1912.

Other Assassination Attempts

In 1932 President-elect Franklin D. Roosevelt was the intended target of an assassination attempt in Miami, Florida. Five shots were fired at Roosevelt's open motorcade. Four people were injured, and Mayor Anton Cermak of Chicago was killed. Roosevelt was uninjured.

President Gerald Ford was attacked by two different women on separate occasions in 1975. He was unharmed on both instances.

President Andrew Jackson was the first president attacked with the intent to kill (see Chapter 1). He was unharmed when the two pistols used both failed to discharge.

CHAPTER 6

Media and the Modern American Presidency

Dwight D. Eisenhower

The heart attack of Dwight D. Eisenhower in 1955 was a watershed event in the history of presidential health because for the first time there was open access to details of a presidential illness. Only the first 12 hours of this illness are in any dispute.

Eisenhower developed "indigestion" while playing golf on September 23, 1955, in Denver, Colorado. At 2 a.m. the next morning Ike had "the big one." He awoke with "severe chest pain," and his personal physician, Dr. Howard Snyder, a 74-year-old military surgeon, was summoned. Dr. Snyder diagnosed indigestion which "is not serious." But after 12 hours of observing continuing pain at the private home where Eisenhower was staying, Dr. Snyder called for help. An electrocardiogram was done by a consulting cardiologist at the home. The electrocardiogram showed an acute antero-lateral myocardial infarction, a heart attack affecting the front and side walls of the heart muscle. President Eisenhower was assisted down the stairs and transferred by private car to Fitzsimons Army Hospital.

Dr. Snyder later claimed he was immediately suspicious of a heart attack, but delayed the electrocardiogram and hospital transfer until the president was more stable and until he was sure of the diagnosis, so he did not alarm Mrs. Eisenhower or the country unnecessarily.

The facts suggest Dr. Snyder initially misdiagnosed the president's symptoms. In Dr. Snyder's defense, the hospital treatment of acute myocardial infarction (heart attack) was not markedly different from home treatment in the 1950s. There were no coronary care units, no catheterization laboratories, no thrombolytic (clot-dissolving) drugs and no defibrillation for ventricular arrhythmias.[43] When Eisenhower reached the hospital, his prescribed treatment was oxygen, heparin (a clot-preventing but not clot-dissolving drug), morphine for pain, papaverine, a medication used for dilatation of the coronary vessels, and atropine to presumably decrease the risk of arrhythmias. Finally, he was placed at strict bed rest. Papaverine is now considered an ineffective drug and is rarely used. Atropine speeds up the heart rate and is used only if the heart rate is dangerously low. It may extend the area of heart damage if used routinely in patients with heart attacks. Even the administration of morphine, although effective for pain relief, has been found in recent studies to increase the mortality rate when given to heart attack victims.

With instructions from Eisenhower to "tell the whole truth," his administration and medical team supplied full information to the press. Eisenhower was later chagrined to learn his bowel function had been a topic of daily discussion. Dr. Paul Dudley White, a civilian cardiologist often referred to as the "Father of American Cardiology," became the main spokesman for the medical team. He delivered an historic press conference several days after the heart attack where he allayed apprehensions about the president's care and educated the country about the epidemic of coronary artery disease and the pathophysiology of the disease. He implied that heart attack victims could live long and productive lives.[44]

---

43 The 21st century goal in treatment of an acute myocardial infarction, heart attack, is to re-establish blood supply to the heart muscle as rapidly as possible. Most heart attacks are caused by sudden occlusion of one of the coronary arteries due to formation of a blood clot superimposed on the more chronic process of atherosclerosis. Once blood supply ceases, myocardial infarction or permanent heart damage begins. This damage occurs over a six to 12-hour period. If the vessel can be opened, either mechanically by emergent angioplasty or by dissolution of the clot by powerful "blood-thinning" medications called thrombolytics, heart muscle can be preserved and the patient's long-term prognosis improved. A complication of heart attacks is electrical instability of the heart, which can cause sudden, life-threatening arrhythmias. Since the 1960s, heart attack victims have been monitored in Intensive or Coronary Care Units of hospitals where defibrillation, the application of direct current voltage to the chest wall, can be employed to abort life-threatening heart rhythm disturbances. Estimates are 25 percent of heart attack victims may die from heart arrhythmias before reaching the hospital, and many more died of arrhythmias at the hospital in Eisenhower's era when there was no treatment available.

This last statement was important since 1956 was an election year and speculation began almost immediately whether Ike would be physically capable to complete a second term. Even the optimistic Dr. White had to admit that he had never had a post-myocardial infarct patient subjected to the pressures of the American presidency. He indicated the ultimate decision would have to be made by the president.

By all accounts, President Eisenhower had a large heart attack. His electrocardiogram (see footnote 19) was interpreted as an "extensive anterior and lateral wall" injury. Fluoroscopy (continuous X-ray which allows a limited ability to view heart motion) showed cardiomegaly (heart enlargement), akinesis (lack of heart muscle movement or contraction) of the anterior wall of the heart and an outward bulge of the anterior wall consistent with a left ventricular aneurysm.[45] Still, President Eisenhower had an uncomplicated recovery with no heart failure (see footnote 19) or recurrent angina (see footnote 18). His recovery consisted of three weeks of bed rest, an additional four-week hospital stay and a six-week rest at his Gettysburg, Pennsylvania farm.

Fortunately, the demands of the presidency were light during his recovery. Stephen Ambrose, an Eisenhower historian, later wrote, "If

---

[44] Dr. White's own study, a 10-year follow-up of patients surviving one month after the initial heart attack, published in 1941, showed a five-year survival of only 49 percent. So by the best data available, it was far from certain Eisenhower would survive a second term. Dr. White, who for years had endorsed activity and rejected invalidism of patients post-myocardial infarction, realized that to a large extent his credibility rested with the clinical outcome of one patient, the president.

[45] Eisenhower died March 28, 1969, nearly 14 years after the heart attack which occurred during his presidency. At postmortem examination, the physicians confirmed severe atherosclerosis of all the coronary arteries. The left anterior descending artery, the vessel that supplies the front or anterior wall of the heart muscle and the anatomic area of Eisenhower's 1955 heart attack, was totally occluded. An occlusion in the proximal left anterior descending artery is often referred to as the "widow-maker" lesion because this vessel supplies a large portion of the overall heart muscle, and heart attacks in this area are often fatal. In Eisenhower's case, this vessel likely occluded and caused the heart attack in 1955. The pathologists also confirmed the presence of a left ventricular aneurysm, first suspected in 1955. There was a large thrombus (blood clot) about the size of a ping-pong ball in this area of the heart chamber. All these findings support the presumption of a large heart attack in 1955.

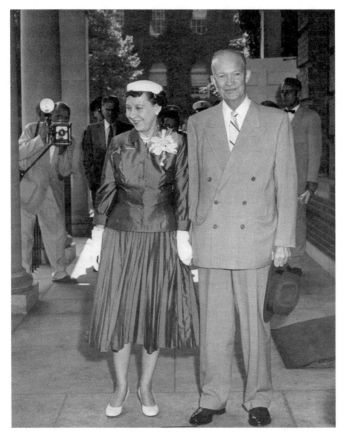

Dwight D. Eisenhower, the 34th president of the United States, shown with his wife, Mamie, leaving the hospital after a 21-day stay for abdominal surgery in 1956 during his campaign for a second term. He became the oldest president to serve during his second term. Courtesy of the Dwight D. Eisenhower Presidential Library.

there was ever a time when the United States in the cold war could get by without a functioning president for a few weeks, it was the fall of 1955."

Initial polls indicated that 80 to 90 percent of press correspondents expected President Eisenhower to retire. But when his recovery progressed without complications, Dr. Snyder paved the way for a second term when he opined that the stress of the presidency may actually be less than the stress of retirement for an intense, ambitious personality

like Eisenhower. So in February 1956, five months after his heart attack, President Eisenhower declared his candidacy for a second term.

The principal issue of the campaign versus Adlai Stevenson was
Eisenhower's health. Stevenson implied the presidency would become a
part-time position and that a vote for Eisenhower may be a vote for vice
presidential candidate Richard Nixon. In a way, the election of 1956
was also a referendum on presidential disclosure of illness. During the
campaign Eisenhower developed a bowel obstruction caused by Crohn's
disease,[46] which required surgery. Pictures at the time of hospital discharge showed a gaunt president *(see above)*.

But after a long presidential history of concealed illness, the unex-
pected occurred in a campaign when presidential illness was disclosed.
The popularity of Eisenhower, the stricken president, soared. Rather
than reject a candidate because of illness, the American public embraced
the candidate. He became more human and sympathetic. The public
wanted him to get better, conquer his illness and continue as their president. Eisenhower won the 1956 presidential election in a landslide.

Unfortunately, Eisenhower's second term was less than successful.
In 1957 he had a small stroke which affected his speech. Although he
had an excellent recovery, he continued to have a mild expressive apha-
sia (difficulty speaking or finding the right words to convey one's
thoughts) throughout the remainder of his life. His administration was
besieged by civil rights issues and cold war tensions. The USSR launched
Sputnik. Historians indicate Ike lost substantial vigor and capacity for
work by the end of his second term. As opposed to previous presidents,
he was not mentally incapacitated, but physically limited. In October of
1960 Eisenhower became the oldest individual to hold the office of
American president. This was later eclipsed by Ronald Reagan.

---

[46] Crohn's disease is a chronic, inflammatory disease of the gastrointestinal system
which most often affects the large bowel and terminal portions of the small bowel.
The cause of this disease remains unknown. Patients often have recurrent bouts of
abdominal pain and diarrhea. Obstruction of the bowel or fistulae, abnormal con-
nections between the loops of bowel, or bowel and bladder, can occur. Although
Eisenhower had a long history of recurrent abdominal symptoms, Crohn's disease
was not diagnosed until characteristic pathologic appearance of this disease was
seen during his abdominal surgery.

If Eisenhower had access to 21st century care, certainly his heart attack could have been limited by either thrombolytics or coronary intervention to rapidly restore blood flow to the heart muscle (see footnote 43). The chance of future vascular events such as his stroke could be significantly reduced by pharmacologic treatments to lower blood pressure and serum cholesterol levels. With his small cerebrovascular accident in 1957 and overall health, many historians believe he was not capable physically of campaigning for Richard Nixon in the 1960 presidential campaign. Nixon lost to John F. Kennedy in a very close election. It is conceivable that a healthy Eisenhower, a popular president, vigorously campaigning for Nixon, could have swung that tightly contested national election to Nixon rather than Kennedy. This writer will leave to your discretion whether an earlier Nixon presidency would have been a blessing or a curse for the country.

The Media Is the Message

In my opinion, the election of 1960 was the last time in presidential history when skeletons related to health issues could safely be hidden in a candidate's closet. The Kennedy/Nixon debates changed the political landscape. In describing the first of those debates, the producer, Don Hewitt, stated, "It's the night politicians looked at television and said, "That's the only way to run for office. And television looked at politicians and saw a bottomless pit of advertising." The media, especially the video media, has developed into a powerful force in American politics. All politicians must manage their media-created image as part of their campaign. Most of a day's campaigning is directed toward creating a "sound byte" that, when run on the evening news, has more overall impact on the campaign because of the masses reached than the delivery of the entire message to the relatively few individuals addressed in person. Politicians use the airways to express their political views in advertisements and debates, but also to cultivate a friendly image on talk shows and private interview formats. Some have even demonstrated their musical talent, or lack thereof, over the national airwaves.

For the media, politics is big business. *Time Magazine* estimated that nearly one and a half billion dollars were spent on media advertising during the fall political campaigns of 2004. Generating interest in

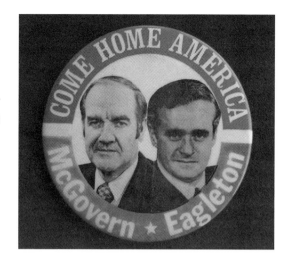

Campaign button of the short-lived McGovern/Eagleton ticket.

politics is good business for the media. Investigative reporting is the result. No longer will the media defer to the office of president or the power of the candidates. No longer will the media allow a president to be out of the public eye for over a year as occurred in the Wilson era. No longer will the media choose to suppress photos showing a disabled or failing president as occurred during the Franklin D. Roosevelt era. Woe to the politician who is not pro-active in revealing health issues.

Consider the presidential campaign of 1972 which matched Richard M. Nixon against George McGovern. McGovern named Senator Thomas Eagleton from Missouri as his running mate.

Several days later, Eagleton revealed to the media that he had been hospitalized in the remote past for nervous exhaustion and had twice received electro-convulsive therapy[47] for depression.

---

[47] The technique of electroconvulsive therapy (ECT), which involves the application of electrical current to the head to induce seizure activity, was introduced in 1938 after observational studies indicated that patients with schizophrenia (psychosis) often had transient improvement in their psychiatric symptoms after a spontaneous seizure. ECT became and remained a common therapy for severe depression at the time of Eagleton's illness. ECT declined in usage after the mid-1970s, presumably due to an unflattering depiction of the technique in the media and the availability of more effective oral antidepressants. However, ECT, now done with the patient under general anesthesia, has increased in frequency in the last decade as a viable and effective treatment for medication-resistant depression.

McGovern initially defended his running mate, stating, "I'm behind him 1,000 percent." But with mounting pressure from the press and the Democratic Party, McGovern changed his mind several days later and asked Eagleton to withdraw from the ticket. McGovern appeared disloyal to some and indecisive to others. He lost to Nixon in a landslide. A clear signal was sent. There are no private health matters if one seeks public office.

If possible, candidates attempt to portray an image of health and a physically active lifestyle. President George W. Bush is not reticent to display his physical fitness by posing for photographs of him jogging or biking. Recent press releases detailed the president's bicycle ride with seven-time Tour de France champion, Lance Armstrong.

Sometimes the media presentation of health can be misleading. During Clinton's White House years he was a jogger, as many stories and photographs attest. This did not prevent coronary artery disease and the need for coronary artery bypass surgery in 2004 at age 58, four years after leaving office. Similarly, pictures of Vice President Al Gore jogging when campaigning for the presidency in 2000 were common. A significant weight gain within months of his defeat casts doubt on adherence to any continuing regular exercise program.

Sometimes the attempts to augment one's media image can backfire. President Carter was an avid jogger. He tried to capitalize on his physical fitness, but the endeavor backfired. He collapsed during a road race in Maryland. Unfortunately, his collapse was photographed and pictures widely distributed (see photo on page 91). The images captured contributed to the public perception that Carter was weak and not in control.[48]

---

[48] Carter needed no additional negative publicity. As his campaign for re-election began in 1980, his administration was besieged by multiple problems. These included the Iranian hostage crisis, where 52 diplomats were seized at the American Embassy in Tehran and held by sympathizers with the revolutionary government of Ayatollah Khomeini, American unemployment exceeding eight percent, skyrocketing oil prices and inflation approaching 20 percent annually. Carter managed to defeat Ted Kennedy for the nomination of the Democratic Party, but lost the general election to Ronald Reagan.

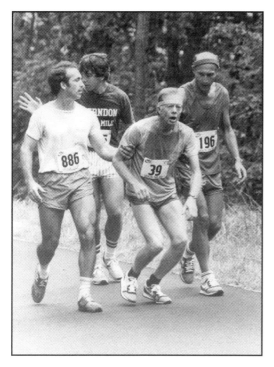

Jimmy Carter, the 40th president of the United States, collapsed during a 10-kilometer race in Maryland. Courtesy of *Running Times,* copyright © Phil Stewart.

It is worth noting that society has changed as well. There is more openness about illness and more acceptance of people with illnesses or disabilities. An aging electorate identifies with candidates with health issues. Still, how the illness is presented to and perceived by the media and public remains important. Here are some examples.

The reporting of the Reagan assassination attempt deserves special mention. The accounts of Reagan's injuries depicted a much less critical scenario than actually existed. Dr. Daniel O'Leary, dean of clinical affairs at George Washington University Medical School, was designated spokesman for the hospital, and a "blackout" was imposed for the remaining health care workers, who were not to communicate with the press. O'Leary's press releases were reviewed by White House staff prior to release. Statements such as "(the president) was never in any serious danger" and "(the bullet was) never close to any vital structure" obfuscated the severity of Reagan's presenting condition. Other statements such as, "He is alert and should be able to make decisions by tomorrow," woefully underestimated the acute disability caused by Reagan's injuries, surgery and necessary narcotic medications for pain. Comments a week later by administrative officials all denied Reagan's disability and can be summarized by, "It's really business as usual," and, "The president will make all the decisions, as he always has." Well-intentioned as it may have been, the hospital and White House personnel obscured the severity of Reagan's illness. The media and the American public were so relieved by the survival of the stricken president that hard questions about the lethality of his injuries and his ability to govern went unasked. Certainly no one within the administration ever questioned Reagan's ability to govern. Although best positioned to determine Reagan's functional status, these same individuals had the most to lose if Reagan was deemed disabled. As Nancy Reagan later said, "There was kind of an unspoken agreement that none of us would let the public know how serious it was and how close we came to losing him."

In 1992 Paul Tsongas ran for the Democratic Party nomination for president. He disclosed a history of lymphoma[49] in 1983, for which he received a bone marrow transplant, one of the early such transplants done in America. He received radiation for recurrent lymphoma localized to an axillary (armpit) lymph node in 1987. But he described himself as "cured" at the initiation of his campaign in 1991. After several early wins in caucuses and primaries, he withdrew as Clinton steamrolled to the nomination. Shortly after the election in 1992, Tsongas had

---

[49] Lymphomas are malignancies (cancer) of lymphoid cells which are usually located in the lymph nodes, the bone marrow and the circulation. Many different types of lymphoma have been identified by the pathologic appearance of the malignant cells. The course of lymphomas can be indolent, with the duration of untreated disease measured in years, to highly aggressive, survival of only weeks if untreated. Bone marrow transplant is a procedure often used to treat highly aggressive lymphomas. Bone marrow aspirates are taken from the healthy donor whose cells are a tissue match for the recipient. The recipient is prepared for transplantation by administration of high dose chemotherapy. In the case of lymphoma, this destroys the patient's cancerous cells and also inhibits the patient's immune response, allowing the donor bone marrow a better chance to establish itself within the recipient. With many cancers, including lymphoma, a disease-free survival of five years after initial diagnosis and treatment indicates a low risk of that cancer ever recurring. However, any recurrence within five years, even with effective treatment for the recurrence, substantially increases the chance of future recurrence and eventual death from the malignancy.

a recurrence of lymphoma and had prolonged hospital stays over the next four years and died a few weeks before completion of the term of office that he sought. Illness was not an issue in his campaign, although he may have been more scrutinized had he won the nomination.

George W. Bush added Dick Cheney to the Republican Party ticket as the vice presidential candidate in 2000 in spite of Cheney's long history of coronary artery disease. He suffered his first heart attack at age 37 and underwent coronary artery bypass surgery in 1988 at age 47. His left ventricular ejection fraction[50] is reported to be 40 percent. A *USA Today* poll during the 2000 presidential campaign showed no effect of Cheney's illness on the presidential election choice. While the election still hung in the balance in Florida, Cheney suffered a small myocardial infarction and underwent coronary angioplasty and coronary artery stent placement. Four months later, he had an "urgent" procedure for re-narrowing of his coronary vessel. In June of 2001 Cheney had an automatic implantable cardiac defibrillator (AICD)[51] placed, which he referred to as a "pacemaker plus," because of an irregular rhythm. Doctors stated that Cheney's prognosis was "terrific" and he returned to work. Very recently he had surgery for resection of bilateral aneurysms (see footnote 34) of the popliteal arteries, which are in the bend of the knee. This is usually caused by atherosclerosis as well. Many may question his politics, but few question his physical ability to perform the duties of vice president.

Senator Paul Wellstone of Minnesota and Democratic Party candi-

---

[50] The ejection fraction refers to the percentage of blood within the heart chamber at the onset of heart contraction that is emptied from the heart with each beat of the heart. A normal left ventricular (main heart-pumping chamber) ejection fraction is 50-70%. An ejection fraction of 40% indicates a mild to moderate reduction in the heart's ability to pump blood.

[51] An automatic implantable cardiac defibrillator (AICD) is a pacemaker type device that can detect life-threatening arrhythmias such as ventricular tachycardia and ventricular fibrillation. If this type of arrhythmia is detected, the pacemaker administers a defibrillation (shock) internally to the heart to restore a normal rhythm. Several studies have indicated improved survival with implantation of AICDs in patients with left ventricular ejection fractions of less than 35%, the population most susceptible to development of life-threatening ventricular arrhythmias.

date Bill Bradbury of Oregon openly have multiple sclerosis. Bradbury often campaigned from a wheelchair. Janet Reno, running for governor of Florida, revealed she has Parkinson's disease. Even the fictional president (played by Martin Sheen) on the television show, "The West Wing," had a health problem — multiple sclerosis.

Currently, the media demands access to the physicians of public officials to obtain medical information. Will the day ever come when media demands the medical records? We can only hope that society's acceptance of disease outpaces the progressive inquisition of public figures.

CHAPTER 7

Cardiovascular Disease, Infections and Cancer and the American Presidency

---

Cardiovascular Disease and Risk Factors

Cardiovascular diseases are the leading cause of death among presidents, which mirrors the general population. Nine presidents have died from heart attacks or complications of heart disease. Six have died from atherosclerotic or hemorrhagic stroke. Over much of the history of the American presidency, factors that increase the development of atherosclerosis were not yet identified. Medical science now has determined that hypertension, high serum cholesterol levels, diabetes, smoking and a history of vascular disease in immediate family members are traits that, when present, increase the risk of an individual developing vascular disease and the consequences of heart attack and stroke. A landmark study showing these relationships was the Framingham study, which was initiated in 1949. The citizens of Framingham, Massachusetts underwent an initial medical history, physical examination and blood work analysis. Subsequent illnesses and diseases occurring over the ensuing 57 years have been observed, recorded and correlated with the initial findings to see what factors predicted an increased risk of future disease. The identification of risk factors has promoted the development of medications to reverse the risky trait such as hypertension or hypercholesterolemia and thus reduce cardiovascular risk. Today medical science has developed medications to lower blood pressure and cholesterol levels. These medications have been proven in multiple scientific studies to lower atherosclerotic events in patients identified at increased risk.

Smoking was epidemic in the middle of the 20th century with nearly 60 percent of adult males indulging in this habit. Although long associated with bronchial irritation, statistical data proving an association between smoking and cardiovascular disease and many forms of cancer did not emerge until the late 1950s to early 1960s. Therefore, it is not surprising that many presidents were smokers. Warren G. Harding, Calvin Coolidge, Dwight D. Eisenhower, Franklin D. Roosevelt and Lyndon B. Johnson were all presidents who were smokers and developed heart disease. Woodrow Wilson died of a cardiovascular cause, specifically a stroke, but did not smoke. Calvin Coolidge died suddenly, five years after leaving office of an apparent heart attack. He was 60 years old. He smoked cigars. Lyndon Johnson is the last president who, at least known to the public, was a smoker. He left office in 1968, 38 years ago. Wilson, Harding and Roosevelt had hypertension in an era before effective antihypertensive therapies were available.

Exercise and maintenance of a normal body weight also decrease the risk of vascular diseases. With this current knowledge of cardiovascular risk factors, many recent presidents have pursued healthy active lifestyles, and most candidates promote at least an image suggesting a physically active lifestyle. President Carter was an avid jogger. President George W. Bush prides himself on physical fitness. He recently changed his aerobic exercise to cycling rather than running to preserve his knees. He also does weight training. He comes by this naturally as his father is a life-long, avid sportsman. Bush, the senior, played varsity baseball at Yale and has remained active over the years with tennis, golf and racquetball. Reagan was a horseman and got his exercise chopping wood. John Kennedy played touch football and golf.

Despite a jogging program, Bill Clinton developed angina and underwent quadruple vessel coronary bypass surgery in 2004. He has a family history of heart disease, mild obesity and admitted non-compliance with diet and medications for hypercholesterolemia. He developed post-pericardiotomy syndrome, inflammation of the membranes surrounding the heart and lung, that occurs occasionally in individuals after chest-opening surgery, and required a surgical procedure for drainage of fluid and removal of scar tissue from around the lung. He now appears fully recovered.

President Lyndon B. Johnson again was a chain smoker. He had a heart attack in 1955, eight years before he became president. He died in

1973 of a second heart attack. There is no record that he participated in regular exercise.

Infections

Infections were often life-threatening in the era before antibiotics. George Washington died of quinsy (pharingitis). The infection caused swelling of his throat, which obstructed his breathing and slowly choked him to death. His doctors exercised liberal blood letting, bleeding Washington to half of his normal blood volume. This also may have contributed to his death. Benjamin Harrison and William Henry Harrison both died of pneumonia in 1901 and 1841, respectively. All these illnesses would likely be cured by antibiotics today.

Although Calvin Coolidge (page 98) died suddenly in his bathroom of a likely heart attack, his life may have been most impacted by the severity of bacterial infection before the discovery of antibiotics. Coolidge assumed the presidency in 1923 upon the death of President Harding. In the summer of 1924 while president, Coolidge's favorite son, Calvin Jr., developed a blister on his toe after playing tennis on the White House grounds with shoes but without socks. The blister became infected and progressed to cellulitis (soft tissue infection) bacteremia, septic shock[52] and the death of young Calvin.

President Coolidge later said, "When he went, the power and the glory of the presidency went with him." Coolidge lost interest in the job of president. Some authors suggest he suffered from a clinical depression. Although he did little on his own behalf, he won re-election in 1924. Although Coolidge's Republican Party controlled both houses, Coolidge remained aloof from Congress and demonstrated no leader-

[52] Bacteremia and septic shock are closely related conditions. Bacteremia indicates infection which has extended from its source to where bacteria contaminate the bloodstream. Once bacteria invade the bloodstream, multiple secondary sites of infection can develop, as can overwhelming, generalized infection. Septic shock, which is abnormally low blood pressure refractory to fluid therapy causing inadequate blood flow to critical internal organs to maintain normal function, often results and may ultimately cause death. Antibiotics treat and cure infection before spread to the blood. Bacteremia, when it occurs, remains a serious infection today, but is still often curable with antibiotics given intravenously, in high dose and over a prolonged course.

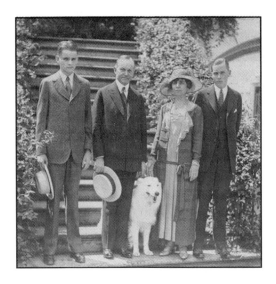

President Coolidge and family posing at the White House in 1924 shortly before son Calvin, Jr. became ill and died. Courtesy of Library of Congress Prints and Photographs.

ship. Historians in 1962 rated Coolidge's presidency 27th among the 31 presidents evaluated.

Cancer

Surprisingly, considering the association between smoking and cancer, malignancies have been relatively rare in American presidents. Ulysses S. Grant is the only deceased president to die due to malignancy. Grant died in 1883, eight years after leaving office, as a result of throat cancer. He died just days after completing his autobiography. He was a heavy cigar smoker throughout most of his life.

Grover Cleveland had successful surgery for oral cancer in 1893 as documented in Chapter 3. Ronald Reagan had part of his colon (large bowel) removed with a cancerous polyp in 1985. He had no spread of disease or recurrence of cancer throughout his lifetime.

There is a suspicion that Franklin D. Roosevelt may have had malignant melanoma. Photographs from 1932 to 1943 show a growing, pigmented skin lesion above the left eye. The lesion is not present in photographs after 1943. The theory is that the skin lesion was malignant and was removed. Some theorists believe that the skin lesion may have represented malignant melanoma, the most deadly form of skin cancer. Speculating further, this cancer may have widely metastasized to other internal organs, causing the weight loss Roosevelt suffered prior to his death. The theory cannot be refuted outright as Roosevelt did not have an autopsy, and his medical records from several admissions to Bethesda Naval Hospital have disappeared. Still considering Dr. Bruenn's account and his constant attendance of Roosevelt in his final two years, a massive intracranial bleed due to hypertension and cardiovascular disease seems the inevitable conclusion of Roosevelt's demise.

CHAPTER 8

Illnesses and the American Vice Presidency

THE CONSTITUTION'S INSTRUCTIONS for presidential succession were ambiguous. Even more unclear was the founder's intentions to fill vacancies in the office of vice president.[53] Twelve times during presidential history the office of vice president has been vacant. Congress attempted to clarify presidential succession in 1947 with passage of the Presidential Succession Act. This established the following order of succession to the president: vice president, Speaker of the House, president pro tempore of the Senate, secretary of state, secretary of treasury, secretary of defense, attorney general, and the various cabinet secretaries in order of creation of the cabinet post held. This legislation did not, however, address the vice presidential position. Up to and including the Lyndon Johnson presidency, no replacement vice presidents were installed following the former vice president ascending to the chief executive position. This fact and deaths in office of the sitting vice president account for the multiple times during history that presidential administrations had unfilled vacancies in the office of vice president.

To address these constitutionally unanswered questions, Congress

---

[53] The Founding Fathers created the office of vice president in the Constitution, but otherwise largely ignored the office. Rather than having a separate election designation, the vice presidential office went to the runner-up in the presidential race. No duties or powers were assigned to the vice president, save presiding over the Senate and casting a deciding vote in the case of tie votes among the senators. No salary was provided by the Constitution or initially by Congress for the vice president. John Adams, the first vice president, wrote, "My country has in its wisdom contrived for me the most insignificant office that was the invention of man ... and as I can do neither good nor evil, I must be borne away by others and meet the common fate." Even today, the duties of the vice president are primarily those assigned to him by the president.

proposed the 25th amendment, and it was ratified in 1967. This amendment fairly clearly outlines presidential succession, filling vice presidential vacancies and also removal of a disabled president from office. The provisions are as follows:

1. The vice president becomes president if the president dies, resigns or is removed from office. This is referred to as the "Tyler provision." It enacts a law which duplicates what has occurred historically upon presidential death as first established by President John Tyler.

2. The president can fill vacancies in the vice presidency. The process to fill a vice presidential vacancy mirrors that of the Supreme Court justices. The president nominates a vice president, who then assumes office upon confirmation by a majority vote of both Houses of Congress. This provision was applied for the first time in 1973 when Richard Nixon nominated Gerald Ford to fill the vice presidential vacancy created when Spiro Agnew resigned in disgrace. Only a year later, Ford became president when Nixon resigned as a result of the Watergate scandal. Ford nominated Nelson Rockefeller as vice president and for the first and only time to date the United States had both a president and vice president appointed to office rather than elected by the American people.

3. The president, recognizing temporary disability, may remove himself temporarily from office with the vice president becoming acting president. This applies primarily to surgeries or anesthetics associated with incapacity of short duration. This provision was employed during Ronald Reagan's colon cancer surgery in 1985. George Bush became "acting president" for just eight hours.[54]

---

[54] Interestingly, the temporary disability provision of the 25th Amendment was not employed during President Reagan's hospitalization following the assassination attempt in 1981 (see Chapter 5). Reagan, with a chest wound, hypotension, anesthesia, surgery and post-surgical pain control, was clearly, temporarily unable to govern. Not only was there no formal transfer of command, but confusion reigned in the White House. Secretary of State Alexander Haig erred constitutionally and politically when he asserted he was "in control." Some suggest this affair indicates

4. In the case of inability or failure of the president to recognize his incapacity to govern, the vice president and a majority of the cabinet can declare presidential disability. The vice president then becomes acting president. Some criticize this provision, an attempt to avoid situations where an impaired president remains in office, such as Woodrow Wilson, as those determining presidential incapacity, the vice president and cabinet secretaries, owe allegiance to the president and therefore may not be objective. However, considering the "watchdog" role of modern American media, the 25h Amendment appears to adequately address presidential and vice presidential succession and disability.

---

that the 25th Amendment, although a major clarification of the Constitution, still may not address all situations of presidential health crises, especially in a nuclear world where foreign affairs can change drastically and instantaneously.

CHAPTER 9

Miscellaneous Illnesses and the American Presidency

WILLIAM HOWARD TAFT likely suffered from sleep apnea. Taft's weight reached 350 pounds during his presidency. Several biographers suggest he over ate in response to stress during his years as the president. He often fell asleep after meals and during cabinet meetings. He once fell asleep and snored loudly during a friend's funeral. His somnolence was so pronounced his wife Nellie dubbed him "Sleeping Beauty." The constellation of morbid obesity, snoring and pronounced daytime somnolence leaves little doubt that Taft suffered sleep apnea[55] during his presidency.

Taft is the only president to subsequently become chief justice of the Supreme Court. His weight decreased to 250 pounds without the stress of the presidency, and he was a far more vigorous and effective chief

---

[55] The most common cause of sleep apnea is upper airway obstruction, which inhibits or stops air exchange despite efforts to breathe. It occurs most often in moderately or severely obese persons and may be mild to lethal in severity. Obese individuals tend to have upper airway narrowing due to increased thickness of the soft tissues of the mouth and throat. In these individuals the normal relaxation and narrowing of the airway that occurs progressively with deeper levels of sleep leads to obstruction during sleep. Hypoxemia, low oxygen levels in the blood, results when air exchange ceases. When the brain detects hypoxemia, arousal through stimulation of the nervous system occurs. A repetitive cycle of airway obstruction, hypoxia and arousal with gasping or snoring ensues. Daytime drowsiness due to lack of restful sleep often results. Long-term complications include hypertension, heart disease and heart rhythm abnormalities and excessive daytime sleepiness. Many experts blame sleep apnea for the majority of automobile accidents caused by drivers falling asleep behind the wheel.

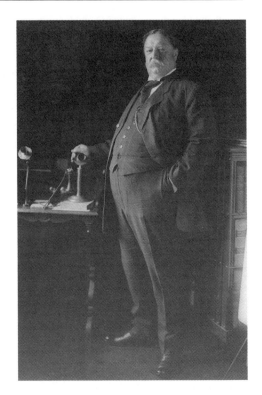

William Howard Taft, the 27th president of the United States, was the heaviest president in American history. Courtesy of Library of Congress Prints and Photographs.

justice than president. Sleep apnea[56] can be weight dependent and may have improved with his weight loss.

Lincoln and Marfan's Syndrome

Over the last 40 years it has been suggested that Lincoln, because of his lanky stature and disproportionately long arms and legs, had Marfan's syndrome. This is a disorder of the connective tissue which often causes dislocation of the eye lens, joint laxity, bone deformity and, most seriously, cardiac manifestations including aortic aneurysm, aortic rupture, aortic valve insufficiency and mitral valve insufficiency.

---

[56] Sleep apnea historically is also referred to as Pickwickian Syndrome. The original case report of sleep apnea published in 1956 recalled a character from The Posthumous Papers of the Pickwick Club, a novel by Charles Dickens published in 1837. Dickens described "a wonderfully fat boy" who repetitively and uncontrollably fell asleep during the day. Dr. C.S. Burwell applied the term Pickwickian Syndrome to the patient he described.

Recently, gene mapping and familial studies have tracked the genetic cause of Marfan's syndrome to several different abnormalities of the long arm of chromosome 15, the gene responsible for fibrillin, a connective tissue protein. Marfan's syndrome may show an autosomal dominant pattern of inheritance in families, which means 50 percent of offspring are affected.

With these new discoveries have come requests from geneticists and researchers for samples of fragments of Lincoln's skull or the clothes of Mrs. Lincoln, stained with her husband's blood, both stored at the National Museum of Health and Medicine, to be utilized for DNA testing.

A special panel was convened to decide whether analysis of President Lincoln's DNA was ethical for historical and medical purposes. Although deemed ethical, it was decided that due to the small amount of Lincoln's genetic material available, the study should be delayed pend-

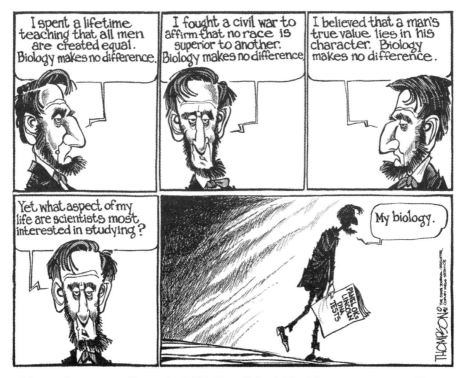

Editorial cartoon, "Lincoln DNA Tests," by Mike Thompson, originally appearing in The State-Journal Register, *Springfield, Illinois, 1991.* Courtesy of Copley News Service

ing improvement in genetic techniques and more complete understanding of the genetic causes of Marfan's syndrome. So the uncertainty regarding Lincoln and Marfan's syndrome continues. Medical experts suggest about a 50 percent chance that Lincoln had Marfan's syndrome. His physical vigor, especially in his younger days, would belie a case of Marfan's syndrome with severe manifestations.

CHAPTER 10

Future Health of the American Presidency

AS DISSIMILAR AS the 42 presidents have been, they still have originated from a narrow segment of the American population. All presidents have been men. They all have been Caucasoid race. All, with the exception of James Buchanan, have been married. Most have been from Protestant religious backgrounds. Most have been lawyers or military heroes. Age at initial inauguration has ranged from John F. Kennedy at age 43 to Ronald Reagan at age 69. So although the office of the presidency is available to most Americans, practically it has been obtainable only by a much smaller demographic. Multiple trends suggest the diversity of this elite presidential group will widen in the 21st century. Two such trends may be related to health.

The Aging of America and the American Presidency

Although the Constitution states a citizen must be 35 years of age or greater to become president, there is no maximum age for the position. Worldwide in developed countries, life expectancy rose dramatically in the 20th century, 71 percent for women and 66 percent for men. The life expectancy of Americans continues to rise. Last estimates in 1998 indicate a mean life expectancy (both men and women combined) of 76.6 years. Recent increases in survival age have been 0.15 years per year or a gain of one-and-a-half years of life expectancy every decade. A healthy 65-year-old can now expect to live to nearly 83 years of age.

The leading cause of death for Americans is no longer acute illness such as infections, but chronic and degenerative diseases of the heart and brain, and multiple forms of cancer. The death rate of patients with heart disease has been halved in the last 20 years by risk factor modification, preventive medications and medical treatment advances.

Smoking has declined significantly in the last 50 years as the health detriments became evident. Obesity and physical inactivity remain epidemic, but susceptible to improvement by a similar public preventive emphasis.

Although the rate of rise in survival age is slowing, other medical advances may be imminent to further extend life. Elucidation of the human genome allows visualization of a day when an individual's genetic pattern can be determined by simple blood testing and then used to predict to which illnesses he/she may be susceptible. Once this is done, an individual-specific preventive program can be prescribed to ward off future disease. Stem cell research offers the potential for regeneration of functional cells in many of the chronic diseases now causing the vast majority of American deaths.

Americans are not only alive longer, but are also healthy longer. Disability at age 65 decreased in the last 15 years from over 26 percent to less than 20 percent.

The Baby Boomer generation is now approaching 60 years of age. Fertility rates in America have declined. Both factors contribute to an older American public.

In 2000 the percentage of the American population age 65 or older was 12.4 percent. By 2030 this is predicted to increase to 19.6 percent. The elderly represent a large, powerful and growing constituency that is more inclined to vote than the average American citizen. Social Security, Medicare, Medicare drug benefits and elder care will become increasingly important societal issues with political implications. At the same time, there are more elderly, vital, experienced and healthy individuals capable and desirous of political office. In the future, the healthy elderly could functionally perform the duties of president into their ninth decade. The demographics of the Baby Boomer generation have already contributed to 16 years of presidential leadership from members of that generation. Will the aging population prefer candidates with experience and more personal insight to the problems the elderly face? It is not inconceivable that another 16 to 20 years of "Boomer" generation presidencies could result. If so, an American president would hold office into his/her 80s.

Health Issues Regarding a Female President

In colonial times voting rights were reserved for men of property on the supposition that this group would be most astute in electing representatives to govern. Women were not the only segment of society excluded from the political process. Still, with the traditional role of parenting and the health disadvantages women faced, political activism would have been impractical during colonial times. The risk of maternal death during delivery, attended by relatives or a midwife with no anesthesia, sterility, parenteral fluids or antibiotics, was in the range of one to one and a half percent. In an age before contraception, fertility rates were high. Mothers averaged five to eight children over their reproductive years. Death in childbirth may have accounted for 10 percent of female mortality. Life expectancy for women varied between 28 and 40 years in different populations and probably lagged that of men. The burden of care of motherless children fell to the women remaining. The ratio of young children to young women is estimated to have been two and a half times the ratio of the modern era.

Times have changed. The maternal mortality with delivery currently is approximately seven and a half deaths per 100,000 live births (0.075 percent). The 19th amendment to the Constitution passed in 1920 guaranteed the right to women to vote. The women's liberation movement opened previously closed doors. Occupations and opportunities are now widely available. With the dangers of childbirth minimized and longevity extended, even women who elect homemaking as their primary occupation complete parenting duties and embark, if they so choose, on diverse second careers. Woman now sit on the Supreme Court and occupy offices at every level of government with the exception of the presidency and vice presidency.

Women now outlive men by an average of seven years. Life expectancy is 73 to 74 years for men and 80 years for women. Although the majority of women in America die of cardiovascular causes, women tend to develop those diseases a decade later than men. The survival advantage affects demographics. Fifty-nine percent of the individuals 65 years old and above are women. With more qualified candidates, a gender advantage in the demographic most likely to vote and women's history of competence at every level of government, it is not a question of *if* we will have a woman president of the United States, only *when.*

Epilogue

REVIEW OF THE medical history of the American presidency emphasizes truths worth comment. The first relates to the medical profession. The history of presidential illness emphasizes the astonishing strides the American medical community has made over the last century. Consider the following:

1. Eighty years ago and 60 years ago Presidents Wilson and Franklin Roosevelt died or were disabled by diseases resulting largely from hypertension and atherosclerosis, for which there were no effective pharmacologic treatments. Now effective therapies proven to prolong life are available for individuals afflicted with hypertension or risk factors for atherosclerosis.
2. Seventy years ago President Harding died of unrecognized and untreated coronary artery disease, congestive heart failure and sudden cardiac death. Medicine now has a plethora of diagnostic and therapeutic options, both medical and surgical, for treatment of heart disease.
3. Fifty years ago President Eisenhower was watched at home for the first 12 hours with an acute myocardial infarction rather than directed to the hospital. Although in error, there was little additional treatment that could be administered at hospitals of that time.
4. Just over a century ago Presidents Garfield and McKinley died from injuries because of the limitations of the medical and surgical techniques of their day, injuries from which they would almost certainly survive today. Contrast that with President Reagan, whose life was saved 25 years ago by modern trauma care.

5. Today we have a vice president with significant heart disease
    and nobody seems to question whether he is physically capable
    of performing the duties of that office. Indeed, Vice President
    Cheney is an example of what 21st century medicine has to of-
    fer — a 30-year survival (and counting) with coronary artery
    disease.

American medicine today confronts many legitimate problems. The
negative impressions of American medicine often outweigh the positive
in the public's awareness, as well as that of the medical providers. History demonstrates, however, that American medicine supplies a level of
care vastly superior to only a decade ago and absolutely undreamed of a
century ago. Previously fatal diseases can now be routinely treated, if
not cured. These improved outcomes soon become expected, and often
the effort and success of medical science in achieving these advances is
overlooked and under-appreciated. Medicine sits on the threshold of
advances that even health care providers may not comprehend. American medicine can be justifiably proud, but not arrogant. Providers and
patients alike are fortunate to live in the medical era we do. History
provides us all a basis for optimism, not pessimism, in the future of
American medicine.

A second impression relates to our government. American history
tends to emphasize the importance of the American presidency. The president gets the credit when times are good and receives blame when times
are bad. We have had many great presidents; some have obtained saint-
hood in the eyes of the American people. The medical history of the
American presidency emphasizes other times when, because of illness,
the presidency functioned less well. But even at periods of presidential
dysfunction, the United States government has continued to operate ef-
ficiently. Why is this? Credit goes to our form of government, a government of shared power among the president, Congress and the courts,
and also shared power among the federal, state and local governments.
Therefore, illness of one individual, even the president, does not precipitate governmental crisis. Rather than the presidency, our form of
government is the champion of United States history.

I marvel at the foresight of the Founding Fathers. They were descendants of lower-class citizens of England and Europe who chose a peril-ous ocean voyage and uncertain life in the New World to their limited prospects in the Old World. These ordinary men did an extraordinary thing. They created a new form of government, a representative repub-lic, where government was by consent of the people governed. The con-cept created a system which has survived and thrived to this day. A gov-ernment that was initially constructed for 13 Atlantic coastal states now equally applies to a country stretching from sea to shining sea.

After this study of the medical history of the American presidency, I find I am less concerned with who is elected, as I have a more abiding faith that our government, with its multiple checks and balances, will ultimately find the path best for the country. History promotes confi-dence and trust in our future and again provides a basis for optimism, not pessimism.

This may be difficult to believe after the 2004 presidential cam-paign and political process. With the allegations, accusations and fabri-cations from both sides, one would think that our political and govern-mental system is dysfunctional and failing. But where the election pro-cess seems to bring out the worst in us as human beings, the post-elec-tion period clearly brings out the best in us as Americans. Senator Kerry stated this most profoundly in his concession speech when he said, "But in an American election there are no losers, because whether our candi-dates are successful, the next morning we all wake up as Americans. And that is the greatest privilege … that can come to us on earth."

My hope for the reader is that this short excursion into the medical history of the American presidency allows the lyrics of Lee Greenwood to always echo true:

" 'Cause there ain't no doubt I love this land;
God bless the USA."

BIBLIOGRAPHY

Books

1. Bumgarner, John R. *The Health of the Presidents: The 41 United States Presidents Through 1993 from a Physician's Point of View.* Jefferson, NC: McFarland & Company, Inc., 1994.
2. Crispell, Kenneth R., and Gomez, Carlos F. *Hidden Illness in the White House.* Durham, NC: Duke University Press, 1988.
3. Ferrell, Robert H. *The Dying President: Franklin D. Roosevelt, 1944-1945.* Columbia, MO: University of Missouri Press, 1998.
4. Ferrell, Robert H. *Ill-advised: Presidential Health and the Public Trust.* Columbia, MO: University of Missouri Press, 1992.
5. Levin, Phyllis L. *Edith and Woodrow.* New York, NY: Simon and Schuster, Inc., 2001.
6. Lasby, Clarence G. *Eisenhower's Heart Attack.* Lawrence, KS: University Press of Kansas, 1997.
7. Remini, Robert Vincent. *The Life of Andrew Jackson.* New York, NY: Harper & Row, 1988.
8. Ackerman, Kenneth D. *Dark Horse: The Surprise Election and Political Murder of James A. Garfield.* New York, NY: Carroll & Graf Publishers, 2003.
9. Abrams, Herbert L. *"The President Has Been Shot": Confusion, Disability, & the 25th Amendment.* Stanford, CA: Stanford University Press, 1994.
10. Gilbert, Robert E. *The Mortal Presidency: Illness and Anguish in the White House.* New York, NY: Fordham University Press, 1998.
11. Degregorio, William A. *The Complete Book of Presidents.* New York, NY: Barricade Books, 1993.
12. Beschloss, Michael. *Illustrated History of The Presidents.* New York, NY: Crown Publishers, 2000.
13. Dallek, Robert. *An Unfinished Life: John F. Kennedy 1917-1963.* Boston, MA: Little, Brown and Company, 2003.
14. Groden, Robert J. *The Killing of a President.* New York, NY: Penguin Group, 1994.
15. Kunhardt, Philip B. et al. *Lincoln.* New York, NY: Random House, 1992.
16. Kunhardt, Philip B. et al. *The American President.* New York, NY: Penguin Putman Inc., 1999.
17. Duffy, John. *From Humors to Medical Science: A History of American Medicine.* Urbana, IL: University of Illinois Press, 1993.
18. Leavitt, J. W., Numbers, R. L. *Sickness and Health in America.* Madison, WI: The University of Wisconsin Press, 1997.
19. Marks, G., Beatty, W. K. *The Story of Medicine in America.* New York, NY: Charles Scribner's Sons, 1973.
20. Vidal, Gore. *Inventing a Nation.* New Haven, CN: Yale University Press, 2003.
21. Hurst, JW., Conti, R., Fye, WB. *Profiles in Cardiology.* Mahwah, NJ: The Foundation for Advances in Medicine and Science, 2003.

22. Ellis, JJ. *His Excellency George Washinton*. New York, NY: Knopf, Borzoi Books, 2004.

23. Kearns, D., *Team of Rivals: The Political Genius of Abraham Lincoln*. New York, NY: Simon & Schuster, 2005.

24. Beers, M.H.; Berkow, R., *The Merck Manual of Diagnosis and Therapy, The 17th Edition*, 1999.

Articles

1. Reyburn, R. The Case of President James A. Garfield: An Abstract of the Clinical History. *American Medicine*. 1901;2:496-501.

2. Gaylord, Harvey D. et al. Death of President McKinley. *J.A.M.A.* 1901;37:779-787.

3. Gaylord, Harvey D. et al. The Official Report on the Case of President McKinley. *J.A.M.A.* 1901;37:1029-1035.

4. Wilbur, RA, Cooper, CM. President Harding's Last Illness: Official Bulletins of Attending Physicians. *J.A.M.A.* 1923;81:603.

5. Nicholas, A, et al. Management of Adreno-cortical Insufficiency During Surgery. *Arch Surg.* 1955;71:737-742.

6. Nichols, J. President Kennedy's Adrenals. *J.A.M.A.* 1967;201:129-130.

7. Foley, WJ. A Bullet and a Bull Moose. *J.A.M.A.* 1969;209:2035-2038.

8. Bruenn, HG. Clinical Notes on the Illness and Death of President Franklin D. Roosevelt. *Ann Intern Med.* 1970;72:579-591.

9. Lattimer, JK. The Wound that Killed Lincoln. *Illinois Medical Journal*. 1970;Nov:514-517.

10. Blinderman, A. Andrew Jackson: The President who would not die conveniently. *NY State Jour Med.* 1972;Feb1:405-412

11. Wecht, CH, Smith, RP. The Medical Evidence in the Assassination of President John F. Kennedy. *Forensic Science.* 1974;3:105-128.

12. Goldsmith, HS. Unanswered Questions in the Death of Franklin D. Roosevelt. *Surg Gyn Ob.* 1979;149:899-908.

13. Massey, EW. Dr. Samuel Mudd: Justice at Last. *South Med Jour.* 1980;73:1375-1376.

14. Brooks, JJ. The Final Diagnosis of President Cleveland's Lesion. *J.A.M.A.* 1980;244:2729.

15. Stevens, RL. A President's Assassination. *J.A.M.A.* 1981;246:1673-1674.

16. Marmor, MF. Wilson, Strokes and Zebras. *N Engl J Med.* 1982;307:528-535.

17. Stokes, SH. A History of Cancer in U. S. Presidents. J Tenn Med Soc. 1987;Jan:13-16.

18. McKusick, VA. Advisory Statement by the Panel on DNA Testing of Abraham Lincoln's Tissue. *Caduceus.* 1991;7:43-7

19. McKusick, VA. The defect in Marfan Syndrome. *Nature.* 1991;352:279-281.

20. Breo, DL. JFK's death—the plain truth from the MDs who did the autopsy. *J.A.M.A.* 1992;267:2794-2803.

21. Breo, DL. JFK's death, part III—Dr. Finck speaks out: "two bullets from the

rear." *J.A.M.A.* 1992;268:1748-1754.

22. Lundberg, GD. Closing the Case in *JAMA* on the John F. Kennedy Autopsy. *J.A.M.A.* 1992;268:1736-1738

23. Various authors. Letters. *J.A.M.A.* 1992;268:1683-1685

24. Carter, J. Presidential Disability and the Twenty-fifth Amendment: A President's Perspective. *J.A.M.A.* 1994;272:1698.

25. Link, AS, Toole, JF. Presidential Disability and the Twenty-fifth Amendment. *J.A.M.A.* 1994;272: 1694-1697.

26. Aaron, BL, Rockoff, D. The Attempted Assassination of President Reagan: Medical Implications and Historical Perspective. *J.A.M.A.* 1994;272:1689-1693.

27. Various authors. Letters. *J.A.M.A.* 1995;274:797-799.

28. Colon, GA. The Bizarre Diseases and Deaths of American Presidents Part I. *J La State Med Soc* 1997;149:147-150.

29. Colon, GA. The Bizarre Diseases and Deaths of American Presidents Part II. *J La State Med Soc.* 1997;149:189-192.

30. Hoang, HM, O'Leary, JP. President Cleveland's Secret Operation. *Am Surg.*1997;63:758-759.

31. Deppisch, LM. Homeopathic medicine and presidential health: Homeopathic influences upon two Ohio presidents. *Pharos.* 1997;Fall:5-10.

32. Deppisch, LM, et al. Andrew Jackson's Exposure to Mercury and Lead: Poisoned President? *J.A.M.A.* 1999;282:569-571.

33. Friedman, WA, Peace, D. A Gunshot Wound to the Head—The Case of Abraham Lincoln. *Surg Neurol* 2000;53:511-515.

34. Colon, GA. President James Garfield's Death: A Criticism. *J La State Med Soc* 2001;153:454-456

35. Public Health and Aging: Trends in Aging—United States and Worldwide. *JAMA.* 2004;289:1371-1373

36. Mokdad, AH, et al. Actual Causes of Death in the United States, 2000. *JAMA.* 2003;291:1238-1245.

37. Fries, JF. Measuring and Monitoring Success in Compressing Morbidity. *Ann Intern Med.* 2003;139:455-459.

38. Cooper, RS, et al. Genomics and Medicine: Distraction, Incremental Progress, or the Dawn of a New Age? *Ann Intern Med.* 2003;138:576-580.

39. Lee, MS, et al. Stem-Cell Transplantation in Myocardial Infarction: A Status Report. *Ann Intern Med.* 2004;140:729-737.

40. Ten, S., et al. Addison's Disease 2001, *J Clin Endocrinal* Metab. 2001; 2909-2922.

Web Sites

1. **www.drzebra.com/prez** Medical History of American Presidents
2. **www.americanpresidents.org** American Presidents: Life Portraits
3. **www.ipl.org/div/potus** POTUS: President of the United States
4. **ap.grolier.com** Grolier Online: The American Presidency
5. **www.whitehouse.gov** The White House

6. **www.lcweb2.loc.gov/ammem/odmdhtml/prespimg.html** Presidential Portraits
7. **www.fdrlibrary.marist.edu** Franklin D. Roosevelt Presidential Library and Museum
8. **www.presidentsusa.net** Presidents of the United States
9. **www.teachpol.tcnj.edu/amer_pol_his/** Images of American Political History
10. **www.cnn.com/2001/HEALTH/06/29/cheney.chronology/index.html** Cheney's History of Heart Problems
11. **www.mult-sclerosis.org/news/Sep2002/USPoliticianwMS.html** A Public Airing of Private Ills
12. **www.ama-assn.org/amednews/1997/amn 97/edit0303.html** Politicians' health: what the public wants to know
13. **www.collphyphil.org/gallrvws.htm** Presidential exhibit reviews
14. **www.healthmedialab.com/html/president/cleveland.html** Grover Cleveland (1885-1889, 1893-1897): The Secret Operation
15. **www.emedicine.com/med/topic2888.htm** Penetrating Head Trauma
16. **www.abrahamlincolnartgallery.com/linklincolnphotographs.htm** Abraham Lincoln Art Gallery
17. **www.suite101.com/print_article.cfm/4996/47901** The Mysterious Death of Warren Harding
18. **www.suite101.com/article.cfm/presidents and first ladies/31466** John Tyler's Presidential Precedent
19. **www.suite101.com/print_article.cfm/4996/30057** William Howard Taft: President and Chief Justice
20. **www.usatrivia.com/pasnatt.html** President Assassination Attempts
21. **www.americanhistory.si.edu/presidency/3d.html** Life and Death in the White House
22. **www.time.com/time/time100/leaders/profile/fdr.html** Franklin Delano Roosevelt
23. **www.cdc.gov/mmwr/preview/mmwrhtml/ss5202a1.htm** Pregnancy-Related Mortality Surveillance — United States, 1991-1999
24. **www.digitalhistory.uh.edu/historyonline/childbirth.cfm** Childbirth in Early America
25. **www.quackwatch.org101 Quackery Related Topics/acego.html** Adrenal Cortical Extract
26. **www.healthmedialab.com/html/president/doctor.html** Medical Care of Our Presidents
27. **www.healthmedialab.com/html/president/roosevelt.html** Franklin Delano Roosevelt (1933-1945) The Daying President
28. **www.weta.org/potomac/history/features/princeton.html** A Twist of Fate (President John Tyler)
29. **www.tech.mit.edu/v112/N61/tsongas.6/w.html** Tsonges Confirms Cancerous Growth

ABOUT THE AUTHOR

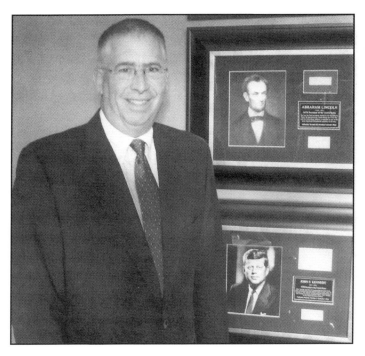

Dr. Jay W. Murphy was born in Canton, Ohio, the home of President William McKinley, and educated in Ohio, a state referred to as the "Mother of Presidents." He graduated from Denison University in Granville, Ohio in 1971 and the Ohio State College of Medicine in 1973. He completed post graduate training in Internal Medicine and Cardiology at the University of Kansas Medical Center. This year he completes 27 years of private practice in Cardiology in the Kansas City area. He currently is the senior partner of Cardiology Services and Director of Preventive Cardiology at Olathe Medical Center in Olathe, Kansas. He speaks widely on preventive cardiology, cardiovascular medications, and function of the vascular endothelium and the Medical History of the American Presidency.

Dr. Murphy enthusiastically combines his medical, cardiovascular and speaking expertise and his love of the American presidency in his presentation, "The Medical History of the American Presidency." For information, please contact him via e-mail at:

jwmrhm@gmail.com